# Hearts Open Wide

by Lily

I remember warm hands
warm, soft, strong hands
gently comforting me, raising me up.
hands holding my hands
as I labored through the night.
and in the quiet dawn hour my son was born.
friends, lover, midwife-doctor there to help re-
    ceive him
and hear his earthly cry.
he was welcomed into our home with warm,
    loving hands.

as I now welcome new, wet beings into this world
with hands warm and loving.
my life has opened wide to embrace the births of
    these new ones.
I feel so honored to answer the holy call of mid-
    wifery,
to help women discover their essence and
    strength as they work
to bring forth new life.
and to watch them welcome their new child.
our hearts open wide to receive them all!
there have been women helping women give
    birth since the beginning
—it will be always—
with our hearts, with our voices, with our hands.

# Hearts
# Open
# Wide

## MIDWIVES
## & BIRTHS

Wingbow Press books are published and distributed by Bookpeople, 2929 Fifth Street, Berkeley, California 94710

Design by Graphic Eye, Berkeley, California
Typesetting by *turnaround*, Berkeley, California
Printed by Consolidated Printers, Berkeley, California

Library of Congress Cataloging-in-Publication Data

Hearts open wide.

   Bibliography: p.
   1. Childbirth—Psychological aspects.    2. Mothers—Biography.
3. Fathers—Biography.    I. Wellish, Pam, 1953-
II. Root, Susan, 1947-
RG658.H43    1987    618.4'092'2    83-32600
ISBN 0-914728-54-7

First Edition: March 1987

*For the Midwives*

# Table of Contents

# Acknowledgement

It was the births of our daughters that made us aware of the uniquely special relationship that exists between a mother-to-be and her midwife and of the selfless dedication of the midwives in our community. We wanted to acknowledge and recognize our midwives and to thank them for truly being with us during our pregnancies as the definition of the word *midwife*, "with women," implies.

Out of our respect and gratitude grew the idea for this book. We asked the women of our community who had given birth with one of the midwives in attendance to write their stories; we planned to present the collection of stories to the midwives as a memento and a tribute to them. But as the stories came in, our idea grew. The stories reflected more than just the dedication of the midwives— they were the stories of strong, wonderful women, women making choices and giving birth in informed, varied and sometimes unusual ways. We began to realize that these stories would have meaning for more women than just those in our community. We began to think that we would have a book for all women interested in birth, a book that conveyed the message that there is more than one choice in how to birth a baby—and that it is *your* choice.

And so it is with heartfelt thanks that we acknowledge all the mothers, fathers, babies and midwives who have made this book an actuality.

# Introduction

The setting for the following birth stories is a rural community in Northern California. The area is isolated and rugged and has always been the home of strong and independent people, from the native Indians to the white settlers and loggers, and more recently the back-to-the-land pioneers. The authors of these stories moved from the cities and urban areas to the seclusion of the countryside, willing to live a life sparse in material wealth but rich in the beauty of the mountains and in harmony with the environment. They were willing to trade the comforts which they had previously taken for granted—paved roads, electricity, telephones, flush toilets—for the physical hardships involved in establishing a self-sufficient lifestyle. They wanted to pursue their idealistic goals: to build their own homes, grow food for their families, provide for their own needs and birth their children in the beds in which they had been conceived.

To simply acknowledge that a woman has a choice regarding where and how she has her baby was to defy the accepted American way of giving birth, labeling these grassroots homebirth advocates rebels against the medical establishment. There was disillusionment with and distrust of the traditional bureaucratic style of medical care that was available; it clashed with the ideals of the newly arrived homesteaders. In order to form a more patient-involved and preventative health care system, the Clinic, which is referred to throughout the following stories and interviews, was established. From its inception in 1976, it has grown from a small medical referral service to a unique family health care facility offering a wide range of medical care, from traditional exams to prenatal yoga and massage therapy.

Simultaneously but separately the age-old art of midwifery was being revived. The initial form it took was simply women helping other women to have the homebirths they desired for their families to the best of their collective ability. Rarely were trained midwives present at births. It became obvious that the women who were attending the homebirths needed to become more formally trained and two of the women undertook that responsibility. Their training enabled them to share their knowledge with other women who wished to apprentice themselves and to practice, with skill, the area of medical care that they loved—assisting women to birth their babies and to help provide the experience these women desired, whether at home or in the hospital.

Inevitably a collective of seven midwives became affiliated with the Clinic and the Clinic's physician, and women of the community were finally able to receive their prenatal care at a place where pregnancy and birth were treated as a joyous event rather than as a disease. But because of the nebulous legal status of lay midwifery and the almost underground nature of homebirths, the association of the Clinic with the lay midwives has always had to be discreet and unofficial. For this reason the name and location of the Clinic have not been disclosed.

With time all things change, and our community has been no exception. The hospital, which ten years ago was not concerned with adjusting to or accommodating a mother's desires, now has a beautiful birthing room that has offered many women an alternative between being at home and having a cold and impersonal hospital birth. The midwives, who at one time were not allowed there, are now welcome to be with women during births. These changes are probably reflective of the changes hospitals all over the United States have undergone as women have articulated their desire for more control over their birth experiences. We rejoice in these changes that have resulted in healthier, happier mothers and babies.

We are pleased that the people who have shared their stories with us are providing other parents with the chance to gain insight into how they have dealt with this passage in their lives. Because it has not been the custom to record the intimate details of birth, we rarely have the opportunity to read birth stories written by our foremothers. It is our ultimate hope that this collection will inspire other mothers and fathers to write the stories of their children's births, to start a new family tradition. The magic of the moment passes like the wind—record it for your children and maybe, someday, theirs.

In motherhood,
Pam and Susan

# PART ONE:
# *Interviews with Midwives*

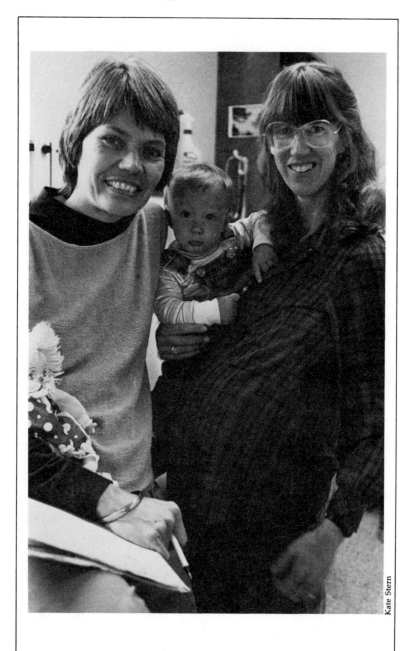

# Kate

Kate became interested in midwifery ten years ago with the birth of her second baby. Her first child, Indigo, had been born in a hospital. "I ended up getting at least two shots of Demerol, that's about as much as I remember, and then the fuzzy feeling of her being born and then not being allowed to see her for twelve hours. The whole experience of not really being aware of Indigo's birth, of feeling like I was the available body they needed, just started gradually over the next couple of years getting me angrier and angrier. So when I became pregnant again I knew right away I wanted to do it at home."

In those days there weren't any midwives in the area, and when Kate asked the doctors at the hospital for help with a homebirth the response was a definite "no." They questioned her right to make such a choice and suggested she not continue receiving her prenatal care from them if a homebirth was what she wanted. By chance she met a doctor who was working with a group of midwives at a birth center seventy-five miles away, and she offered to come and help with the birth. "All of a sudden I felt like I really was going to get what I wanted, that somebody had decided to give me back a little bit of power.

"Sky's birth was beautiful. Two months later I was still floating and writing letters to people about my birth." When Kate found out that training classes for midwives were being offered at the birth center, she eagerly began attending them. "When Sky was about two months old I started going up there one night a week and taking those classes. From then on there was no stopping me—I was just so high."

Within several months she had taken on the role of apprentice midwife. She would go to help a woman in labor while the midwives from the birth center traveled the seventy-five miles. "It really was a sink-or-swim experience for me. Out of the first ten births that I went to, probably four or five ended up happening before the midwives got there. I feel real fortunate that everything went smoothly and nothing heavier happened than what I was able to handle. Looking back now I think, Whoa! Some of the other situations that I've been in, if they had happened then, I wouldn't have been prepared. I really was lucky."

Kate knew that she wanted some kind of official training. Although the direction she first took was to work towards becoming a registered nurse, when she heard about the Physician Assistant Program, she knew it was what she wanted. "I had serious doubts about my being able to work in a nurse's role because I'd had such negative experiences with most doctors, and I'm not real good at taking orders or being told what to do by people I don't have a lot of respect for. The PA is a more independent practitioner and is more involved with general medicine, which was also starting to appeal to me."

Although physician's assistants aren't specifically licensed to deliver babies, Kate saw that there was a policy for extending privileges to cover additional procedures. She knew that if she got through the program, she could probably be licensed to do births. Once in the program, she started talking about what she wanted to do and was allowed to spend extra time working with an obstetrician. She also spent two weeks in the obstetrical ward at a large county hospital.

After completing the PA program, Kate began working at the Clinic as a physician's assistant and continued doing homebirths as a lay midwife. Making the decision to have her license extended for attending normal, vaginal births took her two years. "I was feeling real ambivalent about going through the process of getting legitimate. Part of it was not wanting to let go of the status of lay midwife. I didn't want to make that separation between myself and the other midwives. I was comfortable in the role of lay midwife. Part of it was just seeing the changes that start happening with more medical training. It's so easy to start working from a real fear-oriented place." In her application she didn't specify where she would be doing the births, and since there is nothing in the law saying a PA can't deliver a baby at home, it is legal for her to do homebirths.

Kate recently decided to get hospital privileges to do births there as well as to admit general medical patients in conjunction with Dr. Bill. It wasn't an easy step for her. She had mixed feelings about working in a hospital environment and wondered if there was room in her life for further commitments. "Partly it was just not wanting to go through the red tape and the hassles, and partly it was more of an image problem. It was hard letting go of the image of being a lay midwife who just did homebirths. In the long run I really feel like it's an advantage for all of us, for all the other midwives, for women in the area who want a really wide range of birthing options, because it's one additional possibility—being at the hospital but still having a midwife."

One of the big differences Kate sees between doctors and midwives is that doctors go through a training in which birth is viewed as a potentially hazardous situation. "I'm so glad th PA program is as short as it is because you can easily get sucked into that whole paranoia of looking at everything that can go wrong. For the first year after I got out of training, it was almost like I had lost my intuition. It was hard for me to know where my intuition stopped and my newly acquired medical fears had taken over."

When asked how large a role intuition plays in her work, Kate laughs and says, "A really big one. On a scale of one to ten, probably about six or seven. It plays a bigger part than any of the obvious physical or clinical signs or numbers we've been collecting for the previous nine months."

Kate's conviction is that birth should be a positive, self-empowering experience for a woman. It is her hope that women will gain a sense of self-esteem from their birth experiences rather than lose it. Yet many women whose births don't fulfill their expectations experience a sense of failure and guilt. "There's been such a focus on a successful birth being a vaginal birth, a home delivery or being able to stay in the birthing room—a birth that follows all the expectations and fantasies of this beautiful birth experience. But no matter how the baby is actually delivered, going through the process of pregnancy and labor and acquiring the knowledge to ask questions and make decisions and to find out what the options really are—those are just as powerful a statement. I'd like to see women feeling their personal power in going through the whole thing, regardless of how the birth ends up."

For Kate, being able to help a woman have a good pregnancy and birth experience is a very political act. "My feelings about what pregnancy and birth can be for a woman tie in with my world views and political feelings. It's a way, I think, to help a lot of women see how strong and powerful they can be and maybe help them to take on a little more of that in their personal lives. And I hope that as women become stronger and stronger in their sense of self-worth and self-power, then that's going to start rubbing off on the world in general."

Being a midwife is what Kate really wants to be doing, what she feels she is supposed to be doing. "I still get high every time I'm at a birth, and that high is mostly a sense of awe, of incredible respect for magic and power and strength."

# Lorraine

I don't know how I became interested in midwifery—it seems like it just found me. When I was nineteen, which was nineteen years ago, I went through a pregnancy and birth with a friend of mine. Her family didn't know about it, and she planned to give the baby up for adoption. I got very involved and read the Grantly Dick-Reed book, the only book I found about natural childbirth at that time. I was the "husband" in the husband-coached childbirth but had to sit in the waiting room during the actual birth. That was my introduction to a way of birth in this country—large impersonal hospitals, isolation and powerlessness for those most involved.

After I moved to California a few of my friends had babies, and I went to the hospital with them. One or two had births at home and they went very smoothly. I was lucky and so were they, because I was just breathing with them and reading childbirth books.

When I became pregnant with my son Devlin, I got much more involved in my own pregnancy and decided to have him at home although there was no one around who really knew what to do to help me. During my labor I was surrounded by many people who had never seen a birth but wanted to be supportive. One woman had had a baby so she was the "midwife." At one point when my labor didn't seem to be progressing, everyone became terrified and thought it had gone on too long. So, I was hauled off to the hospital in the back of a van.

We arrived at 4:30 a.m., and the hospital staff was appalled and wanted to do a cesarean section. I had only been in labor about five or six hours, but they were terrified, too. I said I wouldn't sign the consent form unless they gave me oxygen and let me breathe it for a while, then I would reconsider whether to sign or not. I have no idea why I decided to do that, but I was scared, and it gave

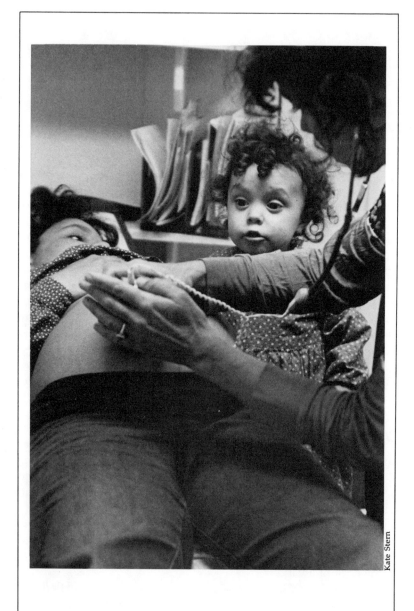

Kate Stern

me something to do and a little space from them. When they came back they said that the baby had to come out. "How?" I asked. I was relieved when they said by forceps. I had been told that the baby would be brain-damaged because they thought I had been pushing all the time that I had been in labor at home, although they didn't explain anything to me at the time. The next day the doctor came in to see me and told me that my baby wasn't brain-damaged.

My birth experience and the reading that I was doing encouraged me to pursue further education in the field of women's health. There was an experimental program training local women in a town seventy miles north of where I lived; Devlin and I traveled there weekly, living out of my station wagon, so I could begin my training. I eventually became a licensed physician's assistant specializing in women's health care. I can legally do perinatal care, but I am still a lay midwife, which is illegal in California. Part of me would like to practice midwifery legally, but legality is not a major issue to me, although I would like to follow with more "hands-on" when I have to transport a woman to the hospital.

My views on birth have grown over the years and there are different factors that have led to that evolution. My medical training is certainly part of it, along with my experience in working with the other midwives and Dr. Bill. But more than anything else I think it's my life experiences, getting older and meeting new people and learning who I am and how other women deal with birth. All the different aspects of my life have been important in my attitude toward birth and what I bring to births.

For most of my life I've been politically involved. Yet, after working in large groups concerned with civil rights, the Vietnam War and nuclear issues, I began to explore the powerlessness I felt in these activities—the overwhelming scale of the fight to bring certain situations to light and the difficulty even to understand what the bases of the problems were and how I could effect any change. When I began working with pregnant women, I felt a coalescence that had never been there in my other involvements. On a small level, very local, very personal, I could help educate and encourage the empowerment of women and of families—encourage them to welcome their child, to nurture it before birth and to call that baby forth through the birth passage into a world which was, at least for that moment, filled with awareness, gentleness and love. I feel very lucky to have found this work.

I think of intuition as one of the creative aspects of medicine and technology. Creativity contributes a whole lot to my midwifery. I think of myself as an artist—not as a doctor. I am often more comfortable with philosophers and artists in terms of whom I relate to and how I approach my work than I am with technicians. I see a real difference between midwives and doctors. Doctors' training is much more technical. Creativity is really wrung out of them during their training. As a group they are much more problem- and fear-oriented because they are dealing not only with birth but with so many other things that require medical intervention. And birth is generally not a problem. Unless the natural process is malfunctioning, doctors aren't needed in aiding normal bodily functions, and basically that's what birth is. As a culture we've been deprived of birth—and death. Once we start sharing that birthing energy with our children so that everyone is exposed to it as a natural, normal function and isn't so frightened of it, then more women will surface as the midwives they are. I feel that being a midwife is an inherent part of many, many women.

I am comfortable with the natural process during a birth. I feel that birth is normal and natural, that women birth the way they live. That's why I like to get to know a woman fairly well before I attend her birth, although it's definitely a personal challenge to walk into the room of someone I don't know and just get into it and deal with it—that's intuition and experience more than anything. My preference in providing good care, and certainly a safe birth, is getting to know a woman and her family fairly well so that I can feel comfortable sensing how she will birth and letting the process take its own course. But I am also very much on it, testing my instincts, listening to the baby's heartbeat, checking the woman's vital signs, and watching. It's very important to do all that, too. I feel like I'm finding a balance between my medical/technical training and my intuition; I'm always learning and changing. Mostly I'm learning to keep out of the way and watch, only entering into the experience if I have a place there.

Communicating, in whatever form seems necessary, is one way to deal with stress, tension and pain during labor. I think sound is a primeval and necessary aspect of human expression, and it often is important in birthing. Touch is also a good way to relieve stress in labor. You can remind a woman that she is holding tension somewhere by touching her in that place. Eye contact or voice contact helps a lot, too. Different women need different approaches or methods. Sometimes women want or need medicines; sometimes those medicines are teas, other times they come through an IV.

I think psychological factors contribute to how a woman births and how she approaches each particular birth experience. Occasionally she has to work through a problem and it helps to have someone facilitate this. As a midwife, I can often predict certain things, but generally I can't intervene during the prenatal course except to explain basic screening principles and try to keep the woman healthy and the baby growing normally. A woman may have a slow labor due to psychological problems, but that might just be the way she has to do it. I feel that sometimes we get too involved in the psychological factors, and I don't think any woman should have to confront everything in her life at the time of her birthing—it just doesn't seem right or fair. Besides, if that were the case, babies might never be born. But occasionally a woman achieves a personal epiphany of sorts when she manages to confront the challenge of birth and the balance of the physical and cerebral powers. When her body works in such harmony with her mind and spirit that she attains an understanding of faith in the birthing process, she can achieve control through letting go.

I'm beginning to see some of the children I helped birth come to the Clinic for birth control, and I think, Oh no! It's been a long time. Maybe someday I'll be helping them birth their babies, but for right now I like the birth control part. I also think having adolescents experience birth in their family—their mother, sister or someone close—having them be there to see the process is one of the best incentives to use birth control there is. I don't think it makes them fearful of sex, but it helps them make connections. My son has been to a lot of births and I feel that it has influenced who he is and his attitudes toward women and life. His respect for life on all levels is phenomenal, it's special; he's a very gentle boy.

As for advice to pregnant women: Eat well, walk a lot or exercise in some way. And try to deal with the fear in your life. Activity helps—if you are in touch with your physical body then you are going to be able to do it more easily. Birth is a physical process, not a cerebral one. Very often that aspect of you, if you are an intellectual, cerebral person, affects your ability to birth; whether that effect is positive or negative depends on how you approach it. But birthing is physical, and you need to be physical too and let it happen.

Each person is different and each birth is different. It's always a miracle when a baby comes out of a woman. It's amazing! I've become very spiritual since I became a midwife, and that was not always my sense of myself or the world; but there is something around, whatever you want to call it, and I definitely feel that power, that life force.

# Kathleen

I became a midwife because of feelings of love, need and anger. The love was for the sacred beauty of birth and birthing women; the need was for service; and the anger was for the cold technological interventionist births that the majority of women and babies are subjected to. I came to midwifery through the high and perfect homebirth of my son, Joaquin.

I am committed to the concept that birth is a natural process the body is meant to carry out and that all women have the power to move through it with grace and strength. But my experiences quickly made it clear that gaining access to that power is difficult for many women. In a culture where sex roles and false hierarchies are disintegrating, most birthing women are left in a position of increasing precariousness, unable to take on the chafing roles our patriarchal culture has imposed on us, yet unable to define the new ones that place us where we can give birth freely.

I feel that I haven't much capacity to change the course of events in an actual labor; I am not an energy weaver. Recognizing this, I have moved away from being a birth attendant and I am giving more and more of my time to prenatal preparation for labor. The tools I bring to pregnant women are yoga and visualization.

A woman in childbirth is a clear distillation of herself. Yoga is one of the most effective ways available to us to hone ourselves for birth. In our culture we rarely meet the concept of positive pain—no wonder so many women flee pain when they meet it in labor. Yoga names pain our teacher and helps us move to a place of strength and self-confidence. To meet the pain and work of labor with a similar ease and confidence is to meet labor successfully.

In addition, yoga strengthens the body. Labor is generally several hours long and aptly named—it *is* hard work. I trained for

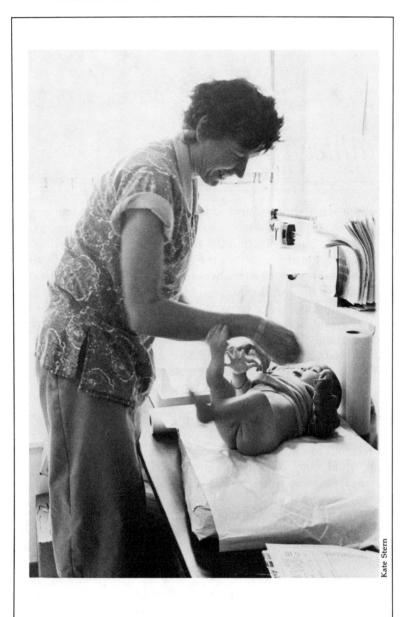

Kate Stern

labor when I was pregnant and encourage other women to do likewise. The combination of muscular strength and breathing for release and peace of mind that yoga can bring are perfect for the work of childbirth. I have never found another discipline that is so tailored for childbirth preparation. Whether with classes or self-practice (but preferably both), I encourage all pregnant women to do yoga.

My other tool is visualization. Bringing women into a light trance state, I guide them through normal, positive labor, with suggestions of finding strength and power to match the power of birth. The concept is that if they are able to enter the visualization and feel what it is like to give birth, even first-time mothers can approach the unknown of labor with confidence. The hope is that women will internalize the imagery and go on to give birth with no problems arising.

We are daughters of a technological age and many of us will need, and be grateful for, medical intervention in our births. Many of us must wrestle with disappointment and even a sense of failure when the birth we have turns out to be so very different from the birth we envisioned. To these women I would say, "Be gentle with yourself." All labors are initiations and all initiations are successful. Love yourselves, love your babes—for these babes, whatever their births, growing in our love, will transform our planet. Our love made manifest, may they manifest peace in our world.

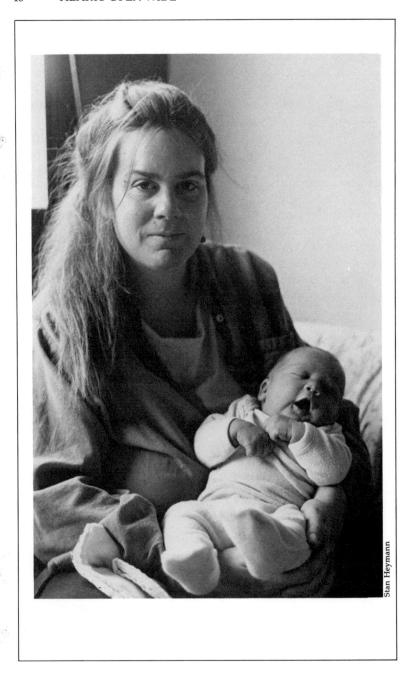

Stan Heymann

# Lily

"I've always liked babies," Lily responds with a smile when asked how she became involved with midwifery. As with many of the other midwives, it was the beautiful homebirth of her son Journey that first opened her heart to the idea of becoming a midwife. When Journey was five months old, Lily helped a friend deliver her baby, and she says, "It grew from there. I don't ever remember thinking, Gee, I really want to be a midwife. It just happened. Something inside me felt it. I'd be at a birth, and I'd know how to do something that I had thought I didn't know. It was there inside, and it just came through."

Lily acquired her midwifery skills empirically. She worked informally with other midwives, but mostly she learned from reading and experience. She studied briefly with a prominent midwife. "She had a class for aspiring midwives. There'd be thirty of us, and all our kids, packed into her living room, sweating, hanging on every word she said. But mainly I learned from just being with other women and midwives, talking with them and exchanging information. And then being at births. I found that every time I was at a birth, everything I'd read or talked about just clicked. I thought there was a lot of grace involved. One of the first births I went to was a breech baby, and I was there all by myself. It was fine, it was perfect, the way most breeches are supposed to be, if you let them be."

Lily recently had her second child, making her the only midwife in the collective to have had a baby after becoming a midwife. "I wish the other midwives would do it too, because it brings you so much closer to birth. It makes you understand what you're doing so much better. I experienced things in my labor that I had *made* women go through in their labors. . . 'I know you don't want to get up and walk, but get up and walk because the baby's head needs to settle,' things like that. Ahh, now I know what it feels like when women say, 'No, I can't do it.' The first birth I went to, a month after Chamisa was born, I realized that everything I said to the woman I could say in all truth and all honesty. I knew just where she was at. It was so fantastic, it made me emotional. I'd be helping her breathe through a contraction that was getting intense, and I'd be getting teary-eyed; I was remembering going through it. I think the emotional connection will fade somewhat, but I hope the essence will stay, because it was the sense of being very much connected to what the mother was feeling and what she needed at the time."

Lily's second labor and birth were much more painful for her than her first birth had been. When asked if there are any techniques she has found useful in helping women deal with pain during labor, she laughs and comments that she can answer from a fresh perspective. "My God, I didn't realize it hurt so much! Ay-yi-yi! I found that all the things I'd been telling women for years to do for the pain didn't really work. . . 'Keep breathing, breathe deeply, breathe deeply, that's it, deep breaths, deep breaths.' Forget the deep breaths! Give me painkillers!"

She goes on to answer the question in a more serious vein. "I've helped a few women who didn't experience pain in their labors and births, they really did not. But I don't know why they didn't. I think it's important to be in tune with your sexuality and with your body, to be really in touch with your mate and to feel good about what he's doing with you. Being alone for part of your labor helps, being completely alone to tune totally into yourself and to realize that you really are doing it all by yourself no matter how many people are there helping you. You need to connect with that grounding place inside yourself. It's hard to do but it's real important."

Although Lily is no longer working at the Clinic, she plans to continue attending births, though not so many as in the past. She mainly wants to help women she has a connection with: her friends, women in her neighborhood, and women whom she has helped with previous babies. "Which is always how I envisioned doing it. Working at the Clinic I got to know women I never would have met or helped otherwise, and that branched out into a whole other thing, attending a lot of hospital births, births that I didn't think I would be doing when I first realized I was getting into this. I learned a lot from it, but I don't need to do that any more. I feel like I need to concentrate on my family, and center on my homestead and my new baby, and maybe another one in a couple of years."

# Rebecca

*How did you come to be a midwife?*

I was raised in a family of medical people—my father, my step-father and my grandfather were all doctors, and I was familiar with the medical world. I went to Guatemala, and while I was there the 1976 earthquake happened. I stood in line to give blood and waited eight hours for someone who knew how to draw blood. During that time I thought, This is ridiculous, I should know how to draw blood by now. So, when I returned to the States I started studying emergency medicine; I learned the basic skills and worked as an Emergency Medical Technician in ambulances. Then I got pregnant with Rosie (who is eight years old now). After Rosie's birth my midwife asked me to help organize some classes to train midwives in exchange for some of the birth fees. I started getting interested in midwifery and sat in on the classes and realized, This is really neat. I ended up going through that series of classes and attended more classes and workshops that were offered. Then I began working with my midwife and later did an apprenticeship with her sister for four years.

*How does the area in which you trained differ from the area in which you now practice?*

It was rural, but not this rural. We always had phones, we were twenty minutes to a half hour from a hospital. It was harder to work there because usually you only had one other midwife you worked with and then your backup physician, so it meant that you had to be on call all the time. Here we have a collective, seven of us, so we can always take an afternoon or weekend off and cover for each other. We have more contact with each other here, and we don't have to worry so much about legal stuff.

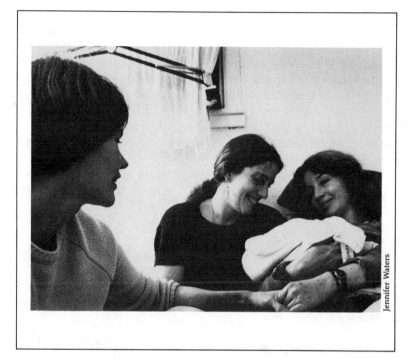

Jennifer Waters

I worked with the Midwifery Advisory Council when Governor Brown was in office. He wanted to see whether it was feasible to initiate a program that would enable lay midwives to become certified. In the beginning the midwives advised the bill writers for the senators in Sacramento. We thought we were going to get a bill that would work for us, but when it went to the first hearing committee the American College of Obstetricians and Gynecologists and the American Medical Association were against it. They had the wording changed so much that the midwives felt that they would be less free than they were without legalization, so we cancelled the bill. We actually ended up lobbying against the bill that we wrote. It doesn't seem likely that lay midwifery will ever be legalized in California, but we're going to keep trying.

The AMA and the obstetricians are threatened; they think that the legalization of midwifery will take away some of their business. Historically they have never wanted women to have power. They don't think that women are competent enough to handle such complicated matters as their own bodies.

*How do you think midwives differ from doctors?*

A midwife is someone who is with a woman from the time they meet to way after she has her baby—the continuity of care is there. A midwife is someone you can call anytime, night or day, and say "I'm scared," and the midwife is going to be there. Midwives are usually women, and they understand the fears, the bodily process, the pain, and everything else about childbirth. A doctor is reassuring on a medical level, but a midwife is there as a sister and a support person, and that's really her main role aside from making sure that the mom and baby are healthy.

With obstetricians birth becomes a management thing—they're very removed. Rarely is there an OB who is really feeling with you—what you're feeling. I must say as a midwife that's one of the harder things, because you really do feel for the woman. When a woman says, "Oh God, I don't want to go to the hospital," and you know that she needs to go, it makes it really hard to say, "You need to go and I've got to take you now." You're a woman, and you remember that feeling. Also, you've created a very close friendship with this woman, and you want to give her what she wants. It's a real hard place to be in.

*Is there anything about actually seeing a baby born that amazes you?*

I haven't quite gotten over the fact that a woman can stretch so much. I always think, This baby isn't going to make it without tearing the mom. But they always do, and I always go away awestruck. The inital awesomeness of birth has passed because I'm so familiar at this point. There is so much going through my mind, so many mechanical things. I don't have time to just sit back and be awestruck. Sometimes I miss that feeling, and I've said to the other midwives that I'd like to go to a birth as a "third" and not be involved, just be there to see what it's like again. You do forget because you are so involved—you're working.

*Have you found any techniques that are useful in helping women deal with pain?*

A tincture of celery seed seems to help, but mainly it's just being there, supporting them, talking them through it, helping them with their breathing. I let them know before labor that it *is* going to be painful and that doing visualization can help.

We also help women learn to take a different attitude: This is going to help my baby be born, instead of, This contraction is hurting me. It's just a different edge on it; it doesn't take away the pain, but it helps women to have control and not feel like victims of their contractions. Occasionally we have to say to a woman in labor, "Hey, you can make this a lot easier on yourself if you just stop the complaining." It's not easy to hear, but women are real receptive during labor, especially when you've developed a good relationship.

*Are there any births you will always remember?*

Oh yeah! There are the ones with really close friends (those have a special meaning) and there are the ones that happen in the car that you can hardly forget.* I think one of my biggest lessons came from a birth I did alone. I had been out of town for about five weeks, and when I got back all the other midwives were booked. There was a woman who had come into the Clinic at thirty-eight weeks gestation. She had planned to do her birth at home alone with her husband but began feeling things weren't right and that maybe she would like to have a midwife there after all. I agreed to do the birth. I did a couple of home visits and she had a nice scene and was a together woman. But it was a birth I would have to walk in to; it was early spring and the roads were muddy. The other midwives kept asking if I felt OK about doing this birth alone. I had never worked births alone, I don't believe it's good, but everyone else was so booked that I just said I'd do it. I was going on faith basically.

When I went to the birth, everything was fine—she had a very quick birth. But when the baby was born he wasn't breathing and didn't have a heart rate, although there had been one right before. I just didn't have enough hands to continue taking the heart tones and deliver the baby, so I had stopped taking the heart tones maybe three minutes before the birth. When there are two of us, one takes the heart tones and taps the beat out to the person delivering and counts out the time. As soon as the baby is born she will call, "One minute, two minutes, three minutes," so you know where you are as far as getting the baby breathing is concerned. Those extra things weren't there, so it was hard. My hands were shaking while I worked. But then the baby gave a big breath, and I'll never forget that. He's a couple of years old now and doing fine. I was glad I was at that birth, because I'm pretty sure he would have died if I wasn't. But I also learned that I will never

*See "On the Road Again," p. 81.

work another birth alone. Your lessons come hard as a lay midwife.

I've seen babies with severe congenital defects, and they are beautiful babies. They teach you a lot in just a few days and then they die. It's painful but the parents grow through it, and you help them. I've only seen one old person die, and the energy of death and birth is exactly the same, a feeling of stillness in the air. The only difference is that as soon as the birth happens there is joy, and as soon as the death happens there's sorrow. But the actual transition—the energy, the awesomeness—is really similar. With birth there is elation and with death grief.

*Do you feel that homebirths are safe?*

Yes, I absolutely believe that home is the safest place to be as long as you have done a good risk screening, have competent backup and aren't too far from the hospital. For sure there are instances when a complication arises that you can't foresee, and in that case there is no comparison to being in a hospital for the technical skill and equipment they offer. But usually you have plenty of time to get to the hospital unless there's a placenta abruptio or prolapsed cord or something like that. Even then sometimes in the hospital they don't have enough time, particularly in a small rural hospital such as ours.

When a woman says she is going to have her baby at home, basically what she is saying is, "I'm going to take control of my birth experience, and I'm going to find someone to help me." I think it's up to the homebirth couple to question the midwife as to how many births she has attended, what kind of experiences she's dealt with, whether she knows how to deal with a hemorrhage, a prolapsed cord. When a woman finds a midwife who is qualified, has doctor backup and good prenatal care, then I think it's perfectly safe.

*Have your feelings or views about birth changed since you first started?*

I used to be a lot more idealistic about it. When you first start as a midwife there is a lot more ego involved—you think, Oh, I'm going to be a midwife and people will look up to me, and that kind of thing. And then you realize that once you are a midwife you're the same old schluck you always were. Actually, you have a hard time with people putting you on a pedestal, looking up to you all the time and assuming that you know all about medicine because you are a midwife, and that's hard. I think what we struggle with now is making people realize that the midwife isn't going to do it for them.

I've noticed that the beginning midwives are a little more enthusiastic; they get crushed if they aren't invited to a birth. The feelings are more intense, and I think that you almost have to have that ego in order to learn, because you have to push through so many barriers just to get the knowledge. To get training as a lay midwife in this country is hard work. It takes years and years of dedication. Also years and years of delivery room doors slammed in your face and nasty doctors talking to you as if you don't know anything. You have to be dedicated, directed and somewhat stubborn to get there.

Now, even if I'm involved with a couple, it doesn't matter if I'm at the birth. It's the care that's important, and it doesn't matter who's giving the care, just that the person is getting it. It's more of a broad vision. I feel like I've seen enough births, and I want to expand into other areas such as working with women before birth with visualization and helping them bring it through in a graceful way, bring the whole family through the prenatal period, the birth and the postpartum adjustment, to being a family. That comes out of my own struggle in becoming a parent. Now I sit down with people in classes, and I tell them, "It's not always fun, it's not always easy, and at times you are going to feel like you hate your kid and all kinds of things, and that's OK." I don't think they believe me at the time, but when those feelings come up they'll remember what I said and not think "I'm crazy" or "What's wrong with me?" When reality hits, it hits really hard, and I'd like to break some myths for new parents before they actually have to go through the changes.

My skill levels have changed. The things that I was interested in seven years ago have changed, and I feel like I know those things well now. I'm interested in the high-risk newborn and high-risk situations because intellectually they're stimulating—I'm pretty scientific-minded.

The emotional and psychological aspects of childbirth are so vast and so necessary, that's a big focus, too. I'm kind of balancing all of it.

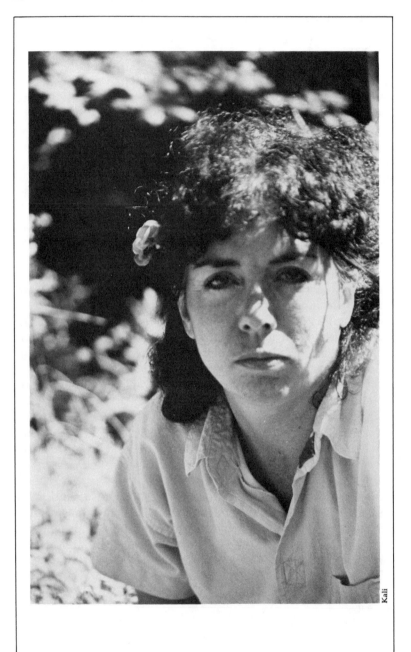

Kali

# Alison

A native of Southern California, Alison moved to the "woods of the Pacific Northwest" when she was twenty-four. After building her own home and giving birth to her second daughter, she began working at the Clinic as a volunteer and training as a lay midwife. When asked what influenced her to become a midwife, Alison related her earliest birth experience—her own. "My mother recently told me how she was anesthetized and how I was delivered from her. When she woke up eighteen hours later, she heard a baby crying in the nursery. She knew it was me—all alone with no one to hold or comfort me. I think that has something to do with my wanting to be a midwife. I'm devoted to the babies. If the mom is unable to take care of the baby right away, I make sure that it gets held and comforted."

The birth of her own children also influenced her. At the age of eighteen she delivered her first child after a very difficult thirty-hour labor. She had wanted a "natural" birth, but what that meant at that time was simply no anesthesia. "Everything else was done according to standard procedure—Demerol, confinement to bed, no food under threat of another enema. It was awful." Her education and awareness of the birth process were very limited. "I thought the baby's umbilical cord was somehow attached to my belly button! When I asked the doctor what was going to happen, he told me, 'Oh, don't worry about a thing. We'll take care of you.'"

Five years later when she conceived her daughter Kali, she was determined to do it differently. "I read tons of books, had a two-hour labor and a homebirth with a midwife. There was such a difference! I *knew* that with support babies could come out a lot easier." Her second daughter, Daymora, was born at home five years later, and Kate was the midwife who "caught" her.

After her homebirth experiences, Alison decided to return to school. "I thought I wanted to go through an RN program, then get a degree as a Family Nurse Practitioner specializing in midwifery." After two years of schooling, she decided that she couldn't balance a seven-year education program and her family. "Seven years of training that was mostly out of my area of focus—it seemed so roundabout. I really wanted to do homebirths, for which my license might be revoked anyway."

The perfect solution for Alison was training with Kate and Lorraine. "This allowed me to be with my daughters and develop my midwifery career at the same time." She is very grateful for this unique situation and feels that the perinatal program at the Clinic could be a model for other medical centers. "But I didn't realize this until I traveled around the United States and talked to women. What we have here is precious, even for California. It's perfect because of the great doctor-midwife relationship, the backup care provided by the doctors, and the way the midwives work together. We all review and discuss the patients we work with, and we all have input and talk about our feelings and insights into things that might not be showing medically."

Alison feels that technically her education has come a long way and that some of her attitudes toward traditional medical practices have changed during the course of her training. "My level of technical expertise has risen, but at the same time it's been important to retain my heart in the matter—my sensitivity and my ability to be intuitive. You can tell when the normal organic process is happening, and you can feel it in the room—there's a harmony, a *cosmic energy* that is happening, and you can take it for granted. You can also tell when something is wrong, you can feel that too. We do a lot of that, just feeling."

When asked if there were any births that she had attended which had a special significance for her, Alison recalled the birth she considers her "coming out party," the first birth she attended without the backup of a senior midwife. "It was the mom's fourth baby, and although it was a simple, very predictable labor, the baby's shoulders got stuck during the delivery and afterwards there was some bleeding. I dealt with those problems and put to use what I had learned—it was awesome to do it by myself. When Kate and Lorraine started as midwives, they were the only ones, they were working on their own. When I started my training, I had them to teach me. It was really hard to take that step from being under their wings to being totally responsible. After that birth I felt real good about myself and everything I'd been taught."

Alison thinks that the training process involved in becoming a rural midwife has to be very thorough. "Women having babies here in the country live so far away from the hospital that the level of responsibility is very different from training in a hospital, where you can turn a problem over to a doctor if you can't deal with it. Here we are responsible from 'A to Z', 'A' being the beginning of the pregnancy, 'Z' being transporting to the hospital if necessary. We are able and willing to accept that responsibility."

When asked her feelings about medical complications and the safety of homebirths, Alison's response was, "There are *no* problems that we are not trained to deal with. How well each midwife does within each of these areas is another thing. But, if it means CPR for the baby all the way to the hospital, we can do it. If it means controlling hemorrhage, that can be dealt with at home, or if there is a need to transport to the hospital, we can use manual compression until we reach assistance. We're pretty capable here, and I'm thankful."

Despite the hardships involved in being a country midwife ("getting up in the middle of the night and driving out muddy roads"), Alison loves her work. "I like babies! They are so wonderful with their unique little souls. I love them. I want to hold them and look into their eyes. Each one is so special." Her enthusiasm remains high for each pregnancy and birth she assists. "The magic of pregnancy is so precious to me. Each family goes through it so few times—it's their own special occurrence. It's a joy and a privilege to be included in this most special passage in a family's life."

# Mary

Mary's involvement with midwifery began when she was twenty-seven after the cesarean birth of her first son Matthew.* She started attending the homebirths of friends and neighbors with a lay midwife and became aware that there were things she could do to help make the birth experience a good one for the mother. "I attended those first births as a breathing coach. I was real good at labor breathing because I had done it myself for two days with my first labor." Feeling useful and being there to see a baby's birth attracted Mary to midwifery.

After the cesarean birth of her second son Nathan**, Mary says, "I changed from being real idealistic about birth, that if you were good and did everything right, you'd have a perfect birth, to the more practical idea that birth is an experience that women go through and sometimes, no matter what they do, the unexpected can happen. I had an enormous amount of disappointment about the birth, and I understand those feelings. I now know that a lot is to be derived from every birth, not by comparing it to some ideal, but by meeting the challenges of your own birth. How you give birth is not a reward or a punishment for having done things right or wrong. The birth itself is significant, but the important thing is that a new person is being born, and that's the miracle."

Mary has worked at the Clinic as a volunteer and childbirth educator. She acquired her training on an informal basis through workshops and as an assistant to the experienced midwives. "My goal is to become a Certified Nurse-Midwife. I realize that I have to go on to a formal education program, and for years now, I've been taking courses in anatomy and physiology, chemistry, micro-

*See "High Expectations," p. 62.
**See "A Second Chance," p. 64.

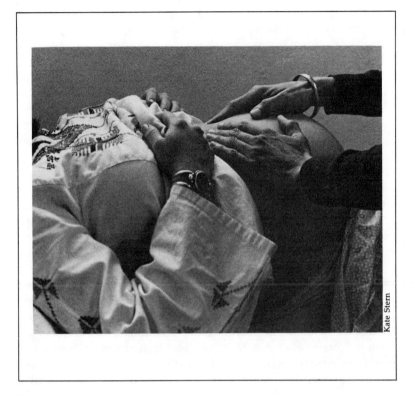

Kate Stern

biology and nutrition. I plan on getting my RN degree through a two-year program; then after one year's experience in obstetrics I can apply for the Certified Nurse-Midwife program which is another eighteen months. So, I'm talking about five years down the road and sometimes that's real discouraging."

Other midwives have commented that the Certified Nurse-Midwife program puts too much emphasis on learning things out of their area of interest and that they can get the same amount of experience in the field; however, Mary says, "That is how I'm different. They are referring to normal births. I already come from a point of view of abnormal births because I've had two c-sections, and I want to be there for women who aren't having normal births—I've been there and I know how it feels. One of my greatest disappointments during my first birth was that as soon as we arrived at the hospital, my midwife and my husband had to leave me. I was there alone, dealing with the medical folks who had never laid eyes on me before, and they were at a loss to help me. I was unable to verbalize, 'Oh God, I'm so terrified!' I was dealing with contractions and being wheeled into surgery—it was overwhelming. I know how that feels, and I know I can help women who are having that experience so they won't feel so scared. And that's important to me."

After achieving her goal to become a nurse-midwife, Mary hopes to work locally. She has seen the local community hospital go through many changes and says, "It now provides a much more humane treatment of people. If you go into the hospital after attempting a homebirth, you will be treated with respect and care, which wasn't always the case. The changes came because of consumer pressure. The birthing room is a fine place to give birth, and it's a great success (economically for the hospital and psychologically for the people who have used it). It offers a nice environment with room for friends, spouse and children. It doesn't look like an ordinary hospital room, and this is comforting, since most people are scared of the medical equipment and are sensitive to a cold atmosphere. The birthing room has wallpaper, flowered curtains and bedspread, a crib, a rocking chair and bean bag pillows which are useful in arranging comfortable positions to labor and give birth in. The mother doesn't have to be shifted from a labor room to a delivery room which is a physically cold environment, suited to medical asepsis and the doctor. Since birth isn't necessarily a medical experience (85 percent of the time there is no need for medical intervention), the birthing room offers a wonderful alternative for people who choose to have their babies in the hospital."

Mary sees her role as a birth attendant gradually changing. "I'm less focused on the delivery itself and more concerned with the preparation of the whole family, including the children. In the future I would like to see clients during their prenatal and postpartum periods. I would like to see how things readjust after the baby is born because I feel that is just as important as the birth. I would also like to teach classes and to work in the hospital and the Clinic. I'm hoping that working as a Certified Nurse-Midwife will fulfill my vocational needs."

# Doctor Bill

My major in college was economics, and I studied health economics. We talked about the doctor shortage, why the price of medical care was so high—those were the kinds of issues we were trying to look at and discuss. I had developed the idea that doctors by and large were...well, "pigs" was the word we used. They were part of the Establishment, fat and greedy, not very caring. It was a popular notion about doctors. I had a theory developed: I thought that the whole training process trained the humanity out of people. In some ways I still think that there is something to it. When I went into medical school, I thought it was going to be hard to go through and come out on the other side with my humane goals intact. If I was going to do that, I was going to have to pursue it actively.

As medical students we were treated with no respect at all. I was treated with more respect when I was in the ninth grade. I wasn't given credit for one original thought; it was just memorization for the first two years, no creative thinking, no questioning. So I just said, "The heck with it, I'm not going to study." I learned to play the fiddle and did other things because I felt it was important to stay in touch. Our medical school class was pass/fail and I made a conscious decision at the start that I wasn't going to try to be at the top of the class—I didn't see what good it would do me. I wanted to go into clinical medicine anyway, not academics or research.

When I rotated through the obstetrical ward as a third-year student, I did deliveries with an intern. I liked it and I found that I could be helpful to laboring mothers. The setting was a big hospital, and a very high percentage of the women were Spanish-speaking, so I had to learn to speak Spanish. I made a special point

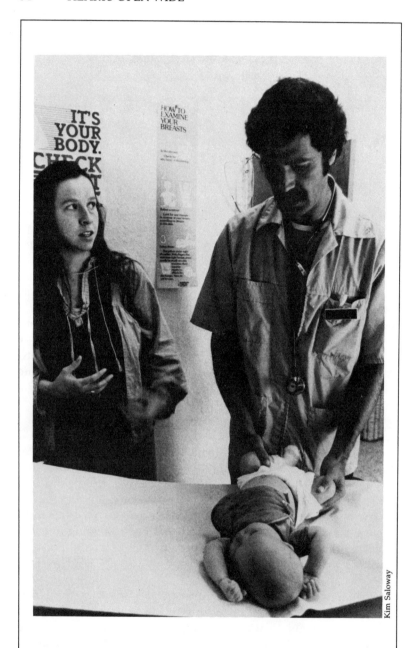

Kim Saloway

to try to make contact with people. It was the thing I was most interested in—I was more interested in the people than in the diseases.

It was very, very busy on the OB ward. I liked it a lot because I could really do something as a third-year student. The interns and residents were often caught up in more complicated things, so if a woman came in at 3:00 a.m., 6 centimeters dilated, it was her fourth baby, and she had had her last one in an hour, they'd call in a third-year student. The interns would show us some things, but they themselves had just learned it the year before; they taught us how to do deliveries and sew up episiotomies but it wasn't like learning from a midwife who had been doing it for twenty years, it was from an intern who was as interested in getting back to bed as anything.

We would try to do a spinal or saddle block anesthesia and use forceps on first-time mothers. I think some doctors actually believed that was a safer way to do it. Another motivating factor might have been to give us practice in using forceps. The mothers were all done up in sterile drapes and put in stirrups; we were all masked and gloved. It was almost like we were trying to pretend that there wasn't really anyone there. But I found that if I questioned everything as I went along—would I want to do it this way, or would I want to be treated this way—I would just get too nuts. It wasn't just in obstetrics; it was everywhere I went. As a matter of fact, OB was a little nicer because it was normal; you had a baby and it was an exciting thing for everybody. I thought it was a gas: It's such a gas, you have to obstruct it an awful lot before you dampen that sense of joy.

The Clinic here fit in with a lot of my ideals: It was community owned and operated, it was created by the consumers, who were consciously trying to achieve a blend of Eastern and Western medical approaches and natural therapies. The fact that I would be working with midwives was played down, and for the first three months I didn't even work with the prenatal program. I had a theoretical fondness for the idea of working with midwives. I was one of the few doctors who did backup for midwives in Sacramento, where homebirths were starting to happen, and I was interested in the idea. By nature I was willing to accept that different things were possible.

The hospital I was working at in Sacramento had a c-section rate of 30 percent, and I was persuaded by the literature that this high rate had to do with people focusing so much on potential problems that they attracted negativity. People worry so much that the tension and tightness slow things down. Most doctors think of pregnancy and birth in a physical, mechanical way; midwives tend to think in an emotional, spiritual way. So I was attracted to the notion of midwives and homebirths.

There are very conscientious and reasonable people who say that it is more dangerous to have your baby at home than in a hospital. It's very difficult to know—the medical data are not clear. There are studies that show both things. I don't object to home-births, but I don't do them for a couple of reasons. The personal reason for me is that I can't bring the equipment to a homebirth that I need to make me feel comfortable. And if I'm not comfortable then I'm not helping the situation. I can't do anything the midwives can't do. As a matter of fact, when it comes to the techniques of perineal massage, dealing with shoulder dystocia and delivering babies without any technological assistance, I think that the mid-wives are probably better at it. I can't do anything special. My particular advantage is having seen a lot of different kinds of complicated births, so if something goes wrong, I can deal with it. I don't see how I could add anything to the home situation—I feel that I might detract if I were nervous. Logistically it's tough, too. When midwives go to a homebirth they spend hours, all day, a couple of days sometimes, and I'm just not into it—I mean I'm into it but I have other things to do. It works much better for me at the hospital because I have nursing backup and other people who are there to help. If I have to go see someone in the emergency room or down the hall, then it's all right there.

The obstetricians in the area think I'm nuts, but they think that for a lot of reasons. I have a different attitude toward money and other things. They are worried about malpractice liability—they think I'm out on a limb. The accusation is that I'm legitimizing the midwives' trip and that if I weren't involved with them, those babies wouldn't be born at home. I don't agree with those assump-tions, and I refuse to worry about being sued—I've got other things to worry about.

When I started working at the Clinic and providing medical support for the midwives, it was a lot clearer because the midwives were helping women to have their babies at home with no medical backup. It was an easy position to defend because the women deserved medical care, and they could make their own choices. I don't say women should have their babies at home—I don't say anything one way or the other. What I say is that it's the mother who decides. I do think people should have medical care. They should have backup, for whatever choices they make.

I also think that if a midwife has a comfortable relationship with a physician, then she will be less hesitant to transport a woman to the hospital in an emergency. I've seen situations where midwives were scared to take someone to the hospital for fear that they or their patients would get in trouble for attempting a homebirth—I wanted to cut into that. Working with the midwives is a way to develop a mutual respect that works better for everybody—we can learn from each other.

When I first began working with the midwives, I sat down with the bunch of them, and they're not lightweights either, and it made me very nervous. I was intimidated by them. So, I carried this big stick—I don't know what it was, a phallic symbol maybe to help me retain my male image. After a year or so when I got to know them better, I could get along without my stick. We've been working together, meeting weekly, for six years. We discuss every case in great detail. There is no prenatal care anywhere that I've ever heard of that's anything like what we do. We don't have that many patients, so we can spend a lot of time and energy on each woman and try to figure out what affects things—attitudes, beliefs, diets, body types, past histories, fantasies, dreams—what makes it so that one lady has a two-hour labor while another has to stay in there for thirty-six hours and ends up with a c-section. And is there a way that we can enter earlier to help ease the process? I've learned a lot from the midwives, and we're learning a lot together.

*Bill graduated from Harvard in 1970 and attended medical school at the University of California at Los Angeles. He completed his three-year residency in Family Practice in 1977 at the University of California at Davis. He then moved to Northern California with his wife to become the Clinic's physician.*

# PART TWO:
## *Birth Stories*

# D'Arcy

## by Elizabeth Montague

For years before she was a reality, my companion David and I talked about our daughter, and we called her D'Arcy. D'Arcy would be our dark-haired, fair-skinned, quiet little daughter. Now that she's here, and I can compare, she's amazingly like the daughter of our dreams.

My pregnancy was normal and healthy—three months of nausea and then smooth sailing. Towards the end, however, my blood pressure was getting higher and higher. I was told that if the pattern continued, a homebirth would be too dangerous. I tried to relax, to rest; truly, I felt fine. I wanted to give birth in the place of my choice, a house that we shared with friends close to the hospital. Our own home would be too far from help should an emergency arise.

Three weeks before my due date I went for my checkup, certain that all would be well. I'd been resting, eating well, and I felt great. Once again my blood pressure was high, higher than ever before. This time I was really discouraged and returned home downcast. As I lay on my couch, dutifully resting and talking to my seven-year-old son Daniel, I wished strongly that I could go into labor early and be spared any further concern.

David was away for a few days on a trip to the city for supplies. I asked him to try to get back early and he returned that night. Ten minutes after he arrived and as we exchanged news, I felt a warm wetness on my drawstring pants. Upon checking, I discovered that I was leaking amniotic fluid, clear and odorless. I caught the next gush and saw a little bloody mucus in the clear fluid. We were all so excited! Labor was imminent, we thought. David packed our birthing kit into the car along with what we needed for a few days at the town-house. The day before I had scoured and scrubbed the designated birthing room, and I was grateful for having done so in advance.

Timing my contractions, I reminded myself that this was early labor, a good time to eat a little, sleep a little, to pace myself. Contractions were irregular, about twelve to eighteen minutes apart with longer pauses. We decided to stay at home for the night

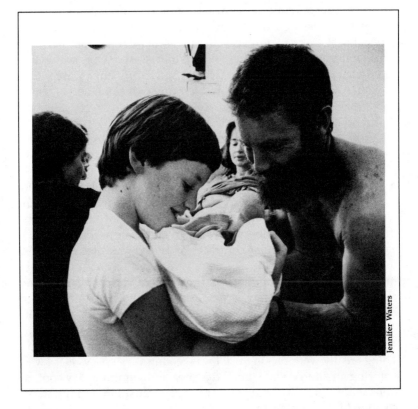

Jennifer Waters

and call the midwives before leaving for the town-house the following day.

The next day, after breakfast, phone calls and a short walk, the three of us set out for town. Contractions were not really regular, but coming steadily every twelve to eighteen minutes. There was no hurry.

It was November 12. A gentle rain was falling as we descended the winding road to town. Suddenly, the sun broke through, and rainbows played over the green hills. My mild contractions were welcome. I felt peacefully at one with this turning of the great wheel, myself lost in this Greater Self. Birthing time lends itself well to such blissful moments and times of vision.

We settled into the birthing room; the fire in the woodstove was crackling while sheets and towels were being sterilized in the oven. Soon my midwife, Becca, arrived to check me. My contractions had stopped though I continued to leak amniotic fluid. All seemed fine except that I needed to get my sluggish labor going because the cervical seal was broken, and there was the danger that infection might enter the womb. Becca told me that most doctors want labor to be well in progress within twenty-four hours after waters have broken. She was encouraging and left me with some herbal teas to drink; she advised me to rest, to eat and not to worry. She said that if all else failed, we would try castor oil.

Another night went by. Contractions began again around 10:00 p.m.; I was delighted and ready to go. Then around 1:00 a.m., they stopped, and I went to sleep. When Becca came by later that morning, I was really discouraged and thought surely I was in for a hospital birth with Pitocin drip, fetal heart monitor and the works. Becca was ever-encouraging; we would try an enema and then castor oil in two doses in order to stimulate a good labor.

I began having regular contractions twelve minutes apart after the enema and castor oil. Big deal, I thought, I'm not going to be fooled into getting hopeful this time. Becca came by and to my relief and delight, she was sure this was the real thing. Upon checking my cervix, she declared that it was 3 centimeters dilated. "Call me when it really gets going," she said and was off again.

For the next hour and a half David and I timed the contractions. Things really were picking up. I was feeling very spacy, as if I were entering an altered state. I had diarrhea and vomiting. My contractions were getting stronger. This feels like transition, I thought, but so soon? I sent David to call Becca. It seemed like ages before he returned, although actually it was about ten minutes. She was surprised to hear from him so quickly and said she would call Kate, the other midwife, a friend who had agreed to photograph the birth, and a doula who was keeping our son Daniel amused throughout this long process.

The contractions were really strong, and I was beginning to have trouble riding the pain. I did my breathing, and it surely helped; gradually I slipped more deeply into a world far away from time. My eyes closed, and my awareness focused on a visualization of my body from the inside: my contracting uterus, my expanding cervix, the small infant moving downward. I told my baby that she was fine, that all was well—not to be afraid. I visualized waterfalls, water rushing through rocky streams, ocean tides ebbing and flowing. Occasionally I surfaced to check on things in the "real world," the world outside my body. Becca had arrived and was checking my cervix. With a glowing smile, she told me I was fully dilated. From 3 to 10 centimeters in less than two hours—I could hardly believe it. More contractions and I returned to my other world. Farther and farther away I drifted, breathing always and moaning through the most painful moments. Moaning seemed to help. People in the room moved quietly so as not to distract me from my work. So many people in a small room, working in harmony as if one organism. David brought a steaming hot wash-cloth at the beginning of each contraction, and we covered my tightly contracting belly with it. It was so comforting.

Pushing contractions now began. The uterus is so amazingly strong, its force is frightening. There were moments of fear and panic, moments when I just wanted to get off this wild ride over which I had no control. I was tired, and I had had enough. Still the contractions came, wave upon wave. I returned to visualization, saw my baby moving down, down the birth canal, centimeter by centimeter. I felt the head descending with each contraction. I reached down and felt the head. Becca checked to see if the cord was wrapped around the neck. It wasn't. I gently stretched my perineum as wide as I could to ease the birth of the head. More pushing, more contractions, and the head was born. With the next contraction came the body—a sweet, tiny girl! So blue, then red; so wrinkled and wise-looking! Such long fingers. One high-pitched shriek and then a quiet, wide-eyed little bundle. There were tears and smiles around the room, and for me, a pretty, healthy daughter and sweet relief. I was starving! Next we enjoyed a dinner of potato-leek soup, red wine, champagne and a chocolate birthday cake. Soon our helpers left, and we four settled down to our first night together. Sleep was delicious after such hard, satisfying work. There beside me, looking peaceful and demure, like a tiny, timeless granny, lay our long-awaited D'Arcy.

*Elizabeth and her family have lived for the past six years in rural California where they have indulged their passions for building, land-scaping and organic gardening. They have recently moved to a larger community to increase the potential of their leather business and to pursue some long-neglected goals and interests: higher education, live music, bicycling and films.*

# Times of Transition

by Jill Duffield

---

I seem to have made some major moves during my two pregnancies. Joseph was conceived in the States, but I spent the first two and a half months of my pregnancy in London, where I was working at the time. I then returned to Dayton, Ohio, where he was born. Benjamin, my second son, was conceived in Ohio, but when I was six months pregnant we moved to the West Coast. Both pregnancies not only signify my sons' new lives but also new starts in my own life. With Joseph, I left behind my country, my family and friends, and to some extent, my career. With Ben, I left behind the carefully built support system for my life as a mother and the wife of a busy family practice resident. In both cases we left behind grandparents who were sad about the prospect of seeing so little of their first grandchildren.

Having a baby in the Midwest usually means a hospital birth; not so with Joseph. My husband Bob's job created a lot of pressure since he worked in a medical world where homebirths were considered unnecessary and probably dangerous. But we resisted and found both a midwife and an obstetrician who gave us support and medical backup. Most of Bob's colleagues chose to ignore the subject of our impending homebirth in order to avoid any confrontation of opinions. But, as the pregnancy progressed, the atmosphere became warmer. There were even jokes about both of us going home from the hospital if I went into labor while there.

It was a hot, sticky and humid summer in Ohio. By the ninth month I was so ready to deliver! I had done everything I possibly could for this child. I'd kept fit, eaten well, taken classes, read every book I could lay my hands on and practiced breathing and relaxation. My due date came and passed. A week later as I was swimming my daily laps at the local pool (by this time swimming was far more comfortable than walking), so many ladies asked, "When's your baby due, dear?" that I got tired of saying, "Last week!"

Finally one afternoon I began to realize that my back ache was taking on a certain rhythm. Connie, my sister-in-law, began to time the frequency, and Loma, our roommate, placed her strong hands on the base of my spine to ease the pressure. So this was labor! I had thought I would feel contractions in my abdomen. My great big belly seemed to do nothing; the ache was all in my back.

Of all times for Bob to be on call! He was at the hospital and was supposed to be working all night. But luckily, another resident agreed to cover for him, and he managed to get home late in the evening. By then I was pacing the floor and needing help to deal with my agonizing back. He checked me, but I was only 2 or 3 centimeters dilated. We paced around together for several hours, but still there was very little progress. Keeping eye contact with Bob through the contractions was a lifesaver, but overall I felt very discouraged. I had read many birth stories telling of the joy and wonder of labor, but this was more like torture.

I had to lie down. Bob and I lay side by side doing the Lamaze breathing together. I was starting to get a little more control, and it seemed like Bob and I were just starting to breathe smoothly together when I noticed his eyes beginning to close. Nights on call at the hospital take their toll on the body!

It was time to call Evelyn, our midwife. She and her two helpers came and quietly set up their equipment while Bob and I lay on

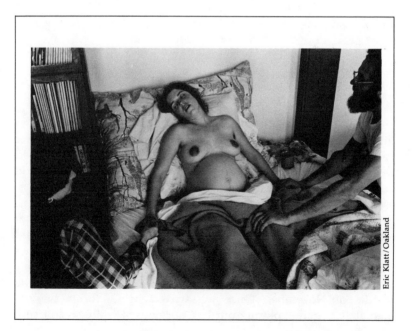

Eric Klatt/Oakland

the bed, now coping quite well with the contractions and their increased intensity. I was beginning to be unaware of my surroundings. I have vague memories of Connie bringing me drinks, or maybe ice. I know Loma took photographs but don't remember her ever being in the room. I focused more and more on my back, deeper and deeper within. This focus was sometimes broken by someone doing something to me, checking my dilation or the fetal heart tone. I became more and more assertive: "Rub here," "Press there," "Hold my leg." I was efficient with my words, to say the least.

At last, in the early morning, my dilation picked up: 4, 5, 7, 8 centimeters. Evelyn broke the amniotic sac, and with a sense of relief I felt the water gush out. I was through transition before I knew it. The books say this is when you get to be angry and cuss people out, but I missed my chance!

I struggled to sit up and hold my knees, getting ready to push. Bob grabbed my hand and held it down so I could feel the baby's emerging head. I almost didn't want to do it. The doctor in Bob took over, and he went to the other end of the bed. I was blowing hard to slow down the pushes. Christina's hair was flying as I blew into her face. Bob quickly unwrapped the cord that was wrapped twice around the baby's neck and began to suction. Another push and the baby was out. Bob lifted him up. "It's a boy," everyone said as he peed all over Bob. No doubt about that!

Hours later this tender, helpless and wonderful infant lay between us as we slept, recovering from our night's work. Our new lives had begun.

❦     ❦     ❦

Ben was different. I felt such a lack of concern and interest in this second pregnancy. I was moving across the country; I didn't have time to be pregnant. The novelty of maternity clothes had worn off. I exercised less and ate a lot. I just hoped it was good quality food; last time I had known it was. People were less interested. Bob didn't talk to the baby in the womb or rub my belly as much. I felt exhausted and somewhat guilty about the lack of attention I was giving this new baby-to-be. Most of all, I had a wild and wonderful two-year-old—how could I possibly love another child as much as I loved my first-born?

We drove across the country in August; Ben was due in the middle of November. Once we arrived in California we immediately began exploring our birth options. I really wasn't sure if I wanted another homebirth. It was ironic, really, that in this area there was almost a reverse pressure to have a homebirth. We had definitely done it the hard way in Ohio. Not that I had any regrets about that decision, but the situation was different here. We were living in a small one-story home that held no strong memories or connections for us. The local hospital looked almost like a small motel and had a comfortable birthing room. Midwives, friends and helpers all seemed welcome, within reason. But most important, my needs and wants were discussed in detail. A hospital birth seemed like an easy choice. I also thought that it would give me a chance to rest and spend time alone with my new baby. That seemed an impossibility at home.

The onset of labor was similar to my first pregnancy: contractions in my back, but they were so gentle that I did not realize what was happening. In the early hours of the morning I was lying in bed, feeling uncomfortable with the usual permanent urge to pee. I was tired of it and complained to Bob. He felt my belly the next time I felt the urge. It was contracting! I decided I should try to sleep the rest of the night, which, predictably, guaranteed I would stay awake.

We got up the next morning as usual, and Bob went to work. The contractions came and went in mild, gentle flows. Sometimes I'd go for half an hour and nothing would happen. A false alarm? Then they would pick up again. I strolled to the grocery store and it was necessary to pause a few times and wait each contraction out. I hoped I would get through the checkout stand without having to pause. My mother had come from England and was staying with us to help in general, but especially with Joseph. In the afternoon we began a game of Scrabble; it was then that the pressure began to quicken. I won the game resoundingly; my mother claimed that she was too concerned about me to concentrate.

By 4:00 p.m. I called Bob for help. He came home, and by 5:00 p.m. we were at the hospital. When Dr. Bill and Kate arrived I was at 3 or 4 centimeters and the contractions were frequent and regular. The next three hours ran together as labor took over my whole body. Everyone seemed to be a tower of strength; Kate, in particular, held on to my back the whole time. Bob and I moaned and groaned since I had given up my unpracticed breathing techniques. We must have sounded like a farmyard. By 7:30 p.m., when Dr. Bill came back from his supper and checked me, I was completely dilated. I couldn't believe it had happened so soon. The water broke, and I heard someone say it was clear: no meconium. Hearing this gave me more confidence as I struggled into a position to push. Bill guided me into two mighty pushes and out came a beautiful, healthy, big boy.

The next few hours were the biggest contrast to Joseph's birth. With very little perineal damage, I was able to sit up and enjoy my new baby and surroundings straight away. My mother brought Joseph to the hospital—he came in shyly, ready to exchange gifts with his new baby brother. Bill played his banjo, we drank some wine and Kate sang a lullaby. This all seems like the perfect memory to me now. It was midnight by the time we'd made our phone calls, and the party was over. Bob and my new child lay sound asleep next to me. I sat and watched them, still overwhelmed with the excitement of the birth, the relief that it was over and the joy of this new life.

*Jill was born and raised in a small town near London, England. She graduated from the University of Sussex and, after a variety of European travels, taught elementary school for five years. At the age of twenty-eight she went to Dayton, Ohio as part of a teacher-exchange program, where she met Bob. Bob now works at the Clinic as a Family Practice physician. Jill is currently at home with their two boys and finds time to garden, play tennis and attend classes related to elementary education.*

# A Journal for Our Baby Kate

by Willow Rain

---

*September 3*

We are in a tranquil sea together, passing from pregnancy through birth, to life apart. You are quiet and still, wriggling occasionally and in the evenings pushing down.

Yesterday morning as I awoke I felt the first contraction, a girdle of tightness around my lower back and belly. You are in no hurry to be born, and I'm enjoying this time of quiet anticipation. I spend my days resting, reading, making your birth announcement and thinking about a welcoming ceremony for you.

At my prenatal checkup at the Clinic on Wednesday, Lorraine found me to be 80 percent effaced and 1½ centimeters dilated. I felt the top of your head with my fingers. What a thrill! You were very quiet, undisturbed by the probings; your heart rate was its lowest, 124 (it's usually been around 144).

Ted's life has slowed down, and we have been able to take long breaks together, lying quietly in the afternoons, melting into each other.

Summer is unravelling into fall, the days less hot, the nights cooler: a good time to be born. We will be able to go on long walks together and feel the season change.

*September 15*

Already you've been out here with us for eleven days. Slowly we get to know each other. You are content when your needs are met; you smile frequently and hugely. I've been slow to understand your needs on occasion, causing you to cry and get tense. But you are forgiving, and daily your trust in me is growing. You cry upon waking, but I've learned to pick you up and cuddle you, which seems to enable you to deal more calmly with waking.

🐞　　🐞　　🐞

Let me record as best I can our birthing journey:

At midnight on September 3, I'd just finished peeing and was back in bed when I felt a warm burst of water between my legs; I knew you were on your way out. I told Ted, and he said to try to get some more sleep. Then, at 2:00 a.m. the contractions woke me up. They were mild pulling, stretching sensations in my lower belly, coming more or less regularly five to ten minutes apart until 3:40 a.m., when I had a harder one that I needed to breathe through. From then on they came regularly every five minutes. I had a clock beside the bed and checked the timing of each one. I felt very relaxed, calm and centered. The sensations were still mild, requiring concentration and centering but not threatening to unbalance me with intensity.

Ted awoke at 6:30 a.m., and we cuddled and shared. At 7:00 a.m. he decided to go call the midwives from a neighbor's telephone, twenty minutes away. The contractions were coming every three minutes but were still mild and manageable. I couldn't stand or walk very easily, and my belly felt cramped and aching, so I lay quietly in bed. I did manage to make some oatmeal, which tasted good and felt nourishing.

Ted had trouble contacting Kathleen and had to wait for the Clinic to open at 9:00 a.m. so that they could phone for him. He didn't get home until 9:30 a.m. The contractions were still coming regularly every three minutes but with increasing intensity. Ted was cleaning the house, tidying up and getting ready. Then at 10:00 a.m. the contractions got stronger, and I needed help. Ted came and lay beside me, holding me. He helped me clear my breathing when the contractions started and breathed with me until they were over, and then he helped me relax. He cupped his hand over my mouth as I breathed to prevent me from hyperventilating, all the time staying centered and calm, guiding me to be that way too.

Soon after 10:00 a.m., friends arrived; I was barely aware of them as the contractions were occupying me completely. Ted was timing them and was able to tell me when they were nearly over, which gave me great strength and courage. We were quite a team, the three of us, working together to bring you into the world.

At 10:30 a.m. Kathleen and Joanne, a doula, arrived—now our team was complete. They supported the three of us as we journeyed toward each other. Kathleen examined my cervix and found it had dilated assymetrically, leaving a cervical lip which she estimated could take two hours to fully dilate. Already my body wanted to push you, but I couldn't risk doing so.

I'm not certain how many contractions it took to relax the lip,

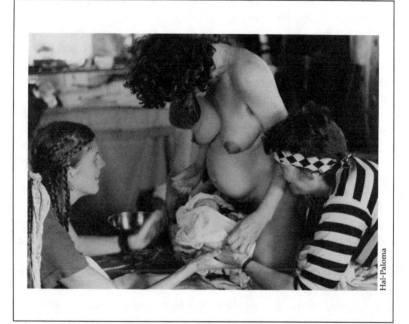

Hal-Paloma

maybe six, but they were the most intense of the whole journey. I was tossing my head and circling my pelvis as you began to move downward. I felt urgent pushings from the middle of my body that I couldn't control. I found it difficult to get into a comfortable position in which to move freely. While I was concentrating on relaxing the lip, my womb began to push you down, and I had to pant so I wouldn't add energy to that pushing. Everything in me wanted to push, but I couldn't let go. I had to stay on top and in control. Kathleen and Joanne helped focus my attention and breathed with me. All of us were caught up in the intensity, rushing headlong. The contractions swept me away. I was swirled in sensations like orgasm, then the energy tide left me, and I was coherent again—clearheaded and able to talk.

I have a very clear memory of Kathleen and Joanne, their eyes full of light, their faces glowing, guiding me, holding me, never leaving me alone. I didn't once feel lonely or abandoned throughout the whole experience, although I had expected to. Ted was behind me most of the time, supporting my back, so I was unable to see his face. But I do remember how he looked when he returned from telephoning—he was radiant, his face and eyes alight with excitement. I love him so dearly.

Finally I asked Kathleen to check my cervix again because the need to push was overwhelming and tearing me apart. When she examined me, she found that the cervical lip was gone and said that she had never seen a lip dissolve so rapidly. The news that I could push was the best I had ever heard.

From then on my memory is a little confused. I was completely taken over by the pushing, and all my strength and energy were focused on you. After four or five pushes—I was on my hands and knees, my body flailing and twirling—Kathleen checked again and saw the tip of your head.

With the next pushes, as I looked through my legs, I saw Ted's hands cradling your head, a memory I hold dear. I didn't see your body come out because I had my head flung back, eyes shut, focusing inward. My womb was pushing you out; I had to stay relaxed and centered. Your whole body came out in a splash of water. I heard you cry as you took your first breath. Then someone said, "It's a girl!"

All wrapped up in a blanket, you were passed forward between my legs, your cord still connecting us, pumping blood and nutrients from the placenta. We waited many minutes for the placenta to empty and the cord to stop throbbing.

I sat back on my heels looking at you. You couldn't open your eyes because of the bright daylight coming in the window behind me, but you were very calm, your hands open, fingers relaxed. Your face was deeply folded, and your ears were flat and slightly misshapen against your head. I couldn't take my eyes off you. You were here—whole, healthy and calm.

The rest of the day is vague and blurry in my memory, though as I write this, what I remember is clear like bright pebbles under a fast flowing stream. You remained calm and peaceful all day and didn't cry until six in the evening when I fed you. You slept all through that first night snuggled in bed beside Ted and me.

The next day a friend cooked supper for us, millet loaf with broccoli. The broccoli made my milk taste bad, and you didn't want to nurse; you cried until you were hoarse. I managed to get some water into you through a straw. What a trial! The following day I ate our placenta cooked with onions and garlic. It was the tastiest meat I have ever eaten.

When Kathleen came back to check on us, she showed me how

to placate you by giving you my little finger to suck. When I told her we'd named you after her, she was moved and thrilled. She felt that we had paid her the highest honor. We had made her happy—a "thank you" for her love and care in bringing you safely into our lives.

*Willow lives with her daughter Kate near the ocean. She is actively involved in land rehabilitation, erosion control and salmon restoration. At her home she has a native plant nursery specializing in perennial bunch grasses which help prevent erosion. She is teaching herself music and makes simple instruments and toys.*

# From Pitocin
# to Midwife

by Jeanne Mattole

Our six children were born in the hospital. My husband would have enjoyed a homebirth each time, but I lacked the faith that all would go right at home. My fears were always for the baby's life. I'm thankful that my husband always supported me completely. He knew my births were rapid and safe and felt we could easily manage a home delivery, but realized my security was what mattered most of all.

Our first child was born in a large university hospital when I was twenty-nine years old. Despite my Lamaze classes, I was very frightened. I phoned the hospital immediately when my water sac broke at 2:00 a.m. When I arrived at the hospital, the nurse invited me to jump right into a bed for a good night's sleep. She said if my contractions did not begin by morning, I'd be given a medication to induce labor; it was feared infection might set in otherwise. I nervously slept until 8:00 a.m., when I was attached to a dripping bottle of Pitocin. Since it was a university hospital, I was assigned a friendly medical student who kept notes of all my activities. Being shy, I didn't enjoy his presence, preferring to be alone with my husband, Mattole.

By evening, after a long and boring day, my contractions were strong and effective. They seemed so strong to me, in fact, that I decided to forego my previous decision to avoid pain medications. I begged for relief and was given a shot of Demerol—it promptly put me to sleep. The next thing I knew, a frantic staff was hurrying me off to the delivery room, patting my face to wake me, yelling "Push! Push!"

Out came our son Donovan. What good news. And then, to sleep. Did I want to hold him? I remember thinking, Oh no! I'm too sleepy. I might drop him. I did hold him briefly—he weighed a ton. I gave him to his daddy and was content to drift off to dreamland.

Since I had rooming-in, my new son joined me immediately. I remember waking and feeling overwhelmed by the awesome responsibility which lay before me in caring for him. The next morning I joined several mothers for a class on bathing babies. So many babies were blond like Donovan. Our matching wristbands did not ease my flitting doubts—Is this baby really mine? I hated the sitz baths I was required to take at shower time because of my stitches. It was a relief to go home at last, that third day.

🐞    🐞    🐞

By the time our second child was due, we were living in the country about twenty miles from the nearest town. Once again I immediately dismissed all suggestions about having a home delivery. We had no vehicle of our own, however, and no immediate neighbors. I wondered how in the world I would get to the hospital. I put my faith in the Lord, and He miraculously provided a ride.

It was a balmy September evening. I'd just gone to sleep when *kerchoo*, I sneezed, and my water sac broke. Not knowing what to do, I lay motionless. An eternity later (or perhaps twenty minutes) my husband came to bed. He'd been at the campfire visiting with an unexpected guest from far away. Immediately he ran to get Bill, our guest, and Bill's car to take me to the hospital. I had to walk from our tipi on the river's edge, across the river to the waiting car. By that time my contractions were coming rapidly. I climbed into the back seat of the VW Bug, and we began the trip to town at breakneck speed. My labor was very strong and I knew the birth was imminent. Our friend thought we should stop and deliver the baby, but Mattole and I wanted to drive on.

When we reached the hospital I was already pushing. The nurses wouldn't let me give birth in the VW back seat as I requested. Rather, Mattole had to lift my uncooperative, very heavy body onto a stretcher so I could be whisked into the delivery room. Fortunately, the nurses knew how to deliver a baby because the doctor arrived only in time to cut the cord. I was wide awake and happy to see our new son—briefly. He was taken to the nursery while I had a good night's sleep. In the morning he was brought to me for an introductory nursing. Thereafter, he visited in my room for nursings and then he was returned to his little crib in the nursery. By the third day I was anxious to take Dylan home and hold him continually.

🐞    🐞    🐞

Our third son came next. At a checkup, my physician pricked my water sac in order to induce labor. He feared I wouldn't make it back to the hospital if my sac broke at home. He was probably right. My labor began immediately, and our Rio was born twenty minutes later. Such an easy delivery! I was happy to send him to the nursery and stay in the hospital the suggested three days in order to rest up before tackling my growing responsibilities.

❦        ❦        ❦

Next came our twins, Morningstar and Meadowlark. This time there was no question of a homebirth since the doctor considered having a baby at my age (thirty-eight) a risk and definitely recommended a hospital delivery with twins.

My water sac broke at breakfast one rainy spring morning. Knowing that my previous labors had been brief, we rushed to get our neighbor to drive us to the hospital. We were in the car and on the go when *whoosh*, we had a flat tire. I'd had no contractions thus far, so I calmly waited while the men frantically replaced the flat tire.

When we reached the hospital, my contractions were slow but steady. There was plenty of time to climb into bed in the labor room, suck ice, and have several sonograms. My labor was no more difficult than my previous ones had been, just slower. By 11:30 a.m., I was ready for the delivery room. We were excited to think that we'd soon know the sexes of our twins. With relative ease, our first little girl popped out. In a quick fifteen minutes she was joined by her sweet sister. Our prayers had been doubly answered with girls, at last. They weighed five pounds each.

Once again, my babies were taken to the nursery to "stabilize" before their first nursing. When one was brought to me four hours later, she turned blue due to loss of body heat. Immediately both girls were placed in matching incubators. The nurses and I fed them bottled formula through holes in the sides. I tried to caress them through the holes, too. Fortunately, I was soon allowed to hold them and nurse them in the warm nursery, and then they were returned to their incubators. Within a couple of days they were sleeping in regular nursery cribs and joining me in my room for nursings. We remained in the hospital a week as I just couldn't emotionally face taking them home before that.

❦        ❦        ❦

Dayspring was to be our sixth and last child. In order to make this delivery extra special, I seriously considered having a homebirth. I enrolled for prenatal care at the Clinic. Previously, all my prenatal care had been at hospitals which had more traditional perspectives towards birthing. I established a pleasant relationship with a wonderful midwife, Alison. She came to my home twice to discuss the coming birth. Since we didn't have a phone, we bought a CB radio. With all the birthing supplies ready, we were in good shape for a homebirth. Still, fears of complications plagued me.

Finally, Mattole and I had a conference with the Clinic's doctor. He said I could expect a safe homebirth because I was in good health and had previously had such easy deliveries. Nevertheless, my advanced age put me in a risk category. He suggested that the decision be based on my comfort and sense of security.

We visited the hospital's brand new birthing room. It did not appeal to me. I decided I'd either have a traditional birth, using the labor and delivery rooms, or I'd have the birth at home. Two days before Dayspring's birth I knew in my heart that it would be another hospital delivery.

On June 16, I woke at daybreak feeling wonderful textbook contractions. Quietly I slid from bed, washed, and woke Mattole. We made arrangements for the care of our sleeping children and jumped into our truck. The day was beginning calmly without a hitch.

Upon reaching the hospital, I entered the labor room and began the usual procedures of birthing—vital signs, enema, hospital gown. Dr. Bill arrived and said the birth would not be soon. He called Alison to keep me company. Mattole was given a hospital breakfast and went out for the morning paper.

Soon Alison arrived with a present of sweet-smelling gardenias from her garden. She suggested I sit up, walk around, and relax. She was so peaceful and supportive—more reassuring and comforting than even my loving husband, as a man, could ever be.

Before long, it was time for the birth. Mattole, Dr. Bill and Alison were all present in the delivery room. I am thankful that Mattole was there as I would have felt lost and abandoned if he were missing at such a special time.

I'd always gained support and comfort from the nurses during previous deliveries; however, Alison's presence was an especially pleasant addition. She rubbed my shoulders, spoke soothingly and demonstrated breathing for me. Dr. Bill was calm and friendly. Together, he, Alison, Mattole and I seemed a team. My pushing was a bit harder than usual because the baby's shoulders were caught. The doctor did some maneuvering which may or may not

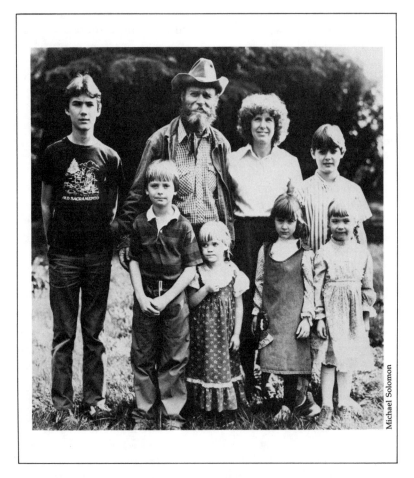

Michael Solomon

have been more stressful at a homebirth. Our new daughter was placed on my tummy, then Alison gave her a wonderful Leboyer bath. Next she was wrapped and taken to my room with me. It was still not yet noon.

Such a joy it was to watch Alison diaper Dayspring for the first time! Then to my breast for her first nursing. We remained together visiting and dozing all afternoon. By 6:00 p.m., baby and I were showing stable vital signs. Dr. Bill agreed that we could go home.

Mattole had shopped during the day so Dayspring and I climbed into a truck loaded with groceries and hay. Home to our family.

Home with a new baby. Home after a long and very special "town day."

❦          ❦          ❦

Although I was helped by my Lamaze classes, the hospital staff, my dear husband and my midwife, the main difference between my first and sixth birth was my own growth toward God. When my first child was born, I was rebelling against the world and had no relationship with God. I took a cute little elf picture to the birthing to "inspire" me—it didn't help at all. At each subsequent birth, my faith and trust in the Lord's ability to care for me grew. I now know the importance of having a personal, prayerful relationship with the Lord. I give Him the glory of our good births.

*Jeanne McCord was born in New York in 1942; Jeanne Mattole was "born again" in California in 1975. She received her BA from Earlham College, Indiana and her Master of Social Work from Hunter College, New York City. She lists her major accomplishments as: teacher, social worker, mother of six, washer of thousands of loads of laundry—by hand, cook of thousands of meals—on a wood stove, ambassador of Jesus, and wife of a horseback evangelist.*

# Doubts Dispelled

by Barbara Sher

---

Not many people were enthusiastic about me having my first baby at home.

"It's too dangerous," warned a doctor.

"You're too old," seconded a nurse.

"You're being naive," fretted a relative.

I was thirty-four and not wise, perhaps, in the ways of infants (I had never changed a diaper); but I knew my mind, and it was made up. I had worked in hospitals before, and I had no romantic notions that "they" would do what was best for me. I had also been on my own a lot and had survived enough situations that I knew I would survive a birth. All I needed, really, was my man at my side.

"It's hippie-witchcraft-bullshit!" shouted my man when I first presented the idea to him as if it were an established fact. He imagined that there I'd be, in a life-threatening situation, none of us knowing what to do, and he would end up driving me at breakneck speed, in the middle of the night, to a hospital. I promised him I would consider his side. I even visited a hospital labor room, but I was as determined as ever. Richard finally resigned himself to the inevitable and to hope—hope that when the first labor pains hit, I'd change my mind.

I had read the few books that were available then on homebirths. Two influenced me: One, a manual for Chinese midwives, was so clear and tidy that it removed some of the unknown fears; the other reduced my fear—it promised that labor pains weren't pains at all, but "pressure." When I told this to my mother, she scoffed and said, "It hurts. A lot!" I believed the book.

Hours into my labor, I believed my mom. But I had been a good student during my pregnancy and had compulsively practiced the yoga relaxation techniques and the Lamaze breathing method. Thank goodness I did, because suddenly I understood their purpose—to give you something to do besides yell "Stop! I want out! I changed my mind!"

Instead I concentrated with all my might on breathing, relaxing my muscles, panting and feeling like a failure. I worried—maybe

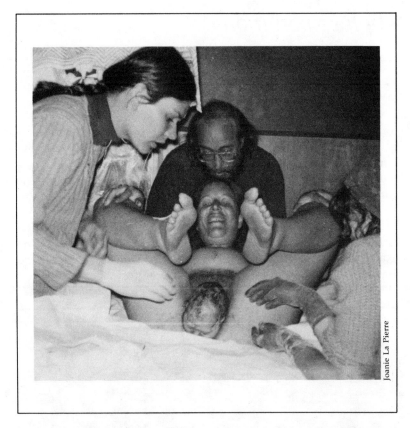

Joanie La Pierre

the book was right; if I were a more "together and enlightened" person, I would feel pressure, not pain—joy, not doubt.

But all doubt dispersed when my baby's head crowned, and it was time (no doubt about it) to push. Oh, what a relief! How in control I felt. What a joy!

As proof of these feelings, I have, in vivid color, a photograph of me, legs apart, with my daughter's head completely out at one end; at the other end, my face with a great huge smile on it. Behind me, propping me up, is Richard, tears of joy on his cheeks.

*Barbara is the mother of two girls and works as an occupational therapist with physically challenged children. She lives with her family in the country in their owner-built home and is the author of the "Homegrown Series," a collection of four books on activities to enrich children's sensory, motor, emotional and mental development.*

# High Expectations

by Mary

I was happy finally to be in labor; I'd been looking forward to it for such a long time—I thought I was six weeks past my due date because of incorrect dates. I was having light contractions, about twenty minutes apart. We went ahead with our errands in town— shopping and laundry—and got home in the early afternoon. The contractions started getting closer together, about ten minutes apart, but still weren't very strong.

After dinner it seemed like things started to pick up. We called Lorraine, our midwife, and Pam, a good friend. When Lorraine examined me, I hadn't dilated very much and the baby's head wasn't engaged. Everyone bedded down for the night, but I

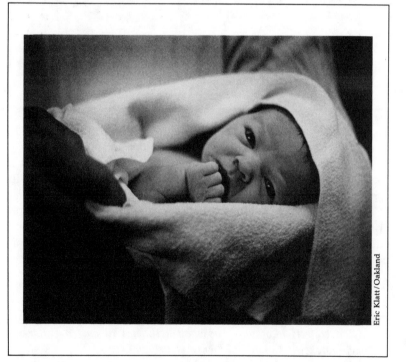

Eric Klatt/Oakland

couldn't sleep. The contractions were about eight to ten minutes apart but strong enough that I needed to do some breathing with them.

I labored all through the following day with the contractions ranging from five to ten minutes apart. I began to have back labor. The most comfortable way for me to handle the pain in my back was to be on my hands and knees with someone putting pressure on my sacrum. My husband Werner and I had some time to ourselves—taking walks, lying out in the sun. It was a warm May day.

Evening fell a second time on my labor, and I was definitely feeling discouraged. It seemed that it would never end, and I wasn't really making progress. Finally there was nothing else we could do but head for the hospital. After a good cry, I resigned myself to giving up my dream of a homebirth.

We got to the local hospital some time after 1:00 a.m. They told me I was just 3 centimeters dilated, and the baby's head was still high. They did an x-ray, which was one of the more difficult moments in my labor. I was left alone for what seemed a very long time. I felt cold, had the shakes and was worried about what was going on. The x-ray showed that there was a large baby's head trying to negotiate a small pelvis from a bad position (posterior). The doctors thought the best course would be to have a cesarean right away. I wasn't ready to give up on having a natural birth, so we arranged to go to a larger hospital and try Pitocin augmentation.

After we made the long drive to the hospital, they hooked me up to the fetal monitor, ruptured my bag of waters, and started the Pitocin. I began having very strong contractions about two minutes apart. After an hour the doctors checked me: I was still 3 centimeters dilated, and the baby's head was still floating. By that time I was ready to see my baby regardless of how it was born. They prepped me for surgery.

I remember lying in the surgery suite looking at unfamiliar eyes, all that I could see of their masked faces. The doctor came over to me and wordlessly held my hand for a reassuring moment. I wanted to be awake for the birth so they gave me an epidural; but because I was so exhausted, it put me in a semi-conscious state. I remember feeling an incredible sensation, an awesome feeling, like the sun coming up—it was my baby being born into the world. They told me it was a boy. He cried loudly right away.

They took my baby to the nursery while the doctor stitched me up. The next thing I remember is being in my hospital room. Werner, Lorraine and Pam were there. They brought the baby in, but I felt so weak and shaky that I was afraid to hold him for fear I'd drop him. They held him close to my face. I was thrilled to see how beautiful and perfect he was—he seemed the most beautiful baby in the world. A few hours later I felt better and was able to hold him and nurse him for the first time. Finally our new life together began.

❧    ❧    ❧

## A SECOND CHANCE

My experience of having Matthew by cesarean birth was very bewildering to me—I had wanted so much to have the perfect homebirth. I really felt incomplete as a woman. I felt that I must have done something wrong and came to the conclusion that it may have been because I was so attached to having a "perfect birth." However questionable that theory was, the failure to live up to my expectations, with the ensuing guilt, caused me a lot of pain. I decided that if I were ever to have a baby again, it wouldn't be for the birth experience but for the baby.

I did become pregnant again. I heard about a birthing center two hours away where they were letting women who'd previously had cesarean sections try for vaginal births. I felt that if the baby were smaller and not posterior, maybe it would fit through my pelvis. I talked to the doctors; although they didn't offer me much hope, they did agree to give me a chance. I felt that even if I didn't give birth vaginally, labor was a worthwhile experience in itself and it was also the best indicator of the baby's readiness to be born. The attitude I adopted was to be neutral and do my best and leave the rest in God's hands. Whatever happened would be OK.

Three days before my due date we took a motel room near the birth center. Two days later I went into labor. This time my contractions were stronger than they had been when I was in labor with Matthew. In the hospital I alternated between resting and walking in the halls. I was having good contractions about five minutes apart. I labored for several hours, but I wasn't making any progress in dilation and the baby's head wasn't engaged. The midwife ruptured my bag of waters, which strengthened the contractions.

During some of the contractions I was starting to have pain in the site of the old incision. It was time to pull out all the stops! The contractions were strong and close together, and it was all I could do to stay on top of them with controlled breathing. Finally I gave in and started moaning. Everyone said it sounded good—it sure felt good. I'd take a deep breath and make a long low moan. After I started doing that, it seemed like the quality of the room and the people in it changed—everyone seemed clear and bright, and we seemed to be transported out of time and space. I was competely at one with my labor, and it felt great.

After a few more hours the doctor checked me—I was 4 centimeters dilated. I felt I'd done my best and was very ready to have my baby out of my belly and into my arms. This time my husband went into surgery with me and held my hand the whole time. I was wide awake for Nathan's birth. They gave the baby to Werner and he brought him over to see me. It was amazing to actually see the baby who had been growing inside me all that time, to see that he wasn't a part of my body but a unique individual.

❦     ❦     ❦

Both of my cesarean births had their good and bad moments. I don't think that having surgery can ever be described as pleasant; but birth, with all its attendant feelings of wonder and joy, is birth, regardless of how it happens.

For a long time after my first birth I had bouts of depression, feeling that I would never be complete, that somehow I just hadn't tried hard enough. Nathan's birth resolved many of those feelings because I had consciously done the best I could. When it all boils down, birth by cesarean is how I experience birth. And it is the coming forth of another human being that is ultimately the important thing, not just the mechanics of how it takes place. Our focus belongs on that new life and on being parents.

*Mary has now completed her first year of a two-year RN program. She plans to work at the local hospital after graduating and hopes to eventually be accepted into a Certified Nurse-Midwife program.*

# Jacob's Birth

by Victoria Shafer

I went to the Clinic throughout my pregnancy, seeing Kate and
Lorraine. Having had Ramona, my second child, at home four
years previously, I wanted to have this baby at home, too. My only
anxiety was that I'd had a retained placenta with Ramona and
Lorraine had to remove it manually, which was quite painful. I was
told that there was a possibility that it could happen again. Kate
and Lorraine were great about explaining the alternatives if this
should happen. After considerable thought, my husband Eric and
I decided to have the baby at home, feeling confident about the
midwives' experience and the equipment they had available for
homebirths.

I had two false labors before the real thing. This was a surprise
to me as I felt I would surely know what to expect by my third
child. One series of contractions was regular for over six hours. I
had all my birth equipment ready, and we called Lorraine at 9:00
p.m.; but by 2:00 a.m., the contractions just faded away. What a
letdown!

So, needless to say, I was overly anxious to give birth when five
days later my water broke at 3:00 a.m. The contractions were mild
and regular, five to ten minutes apart, and I knew that this was the
day. I woke Eric, and he called Lorraine. She arrived at 4:00 a.m.
and checked me. I was a few centimeters dilated and having
contractions five minutes apart. Eric and Lorraine decided to get
some sleep as the birth was not imminent, and I was feeling calm.
I even slept for a half hour.

At 6:30 a.m., Lorraine came in to see how I was doing. I felt
great. My mom and dad were visiting, and Mom was going to
watch the birth with our children, Erica, Ramona, and our foster
son, Stanley. I told Eric that I thought the baby would be born
around noon. I walked around the house talking to Mom and
Lorraine, and using slow deep breathing during contractions. Erica
and Ramona came into the bedroom to see me at 8:30 a.m., and I
talked to them about how I was feeling. Sitting on the edge of the
bed or standing during contractions felt best.

At 9:00 a.m., I needed to concentrate more on my breathing

during the contractions, which were about two to three minutes apart and becoming much stronger. Lorraine checked me, and I was 6 centimeters dilated. She said she could feel the baby's fuzzy hair, which made me feel good. I was able to think about how very soon I would see this little person I had carried for so long. When I concentrated on the joy of that, the contractions didn't seem so bad. I was having back labor, which was painful, but Eric massaged my lower back and Lorraine held my hands. Lots of positive, loving energy and deep, slow breathing were the keys for me.

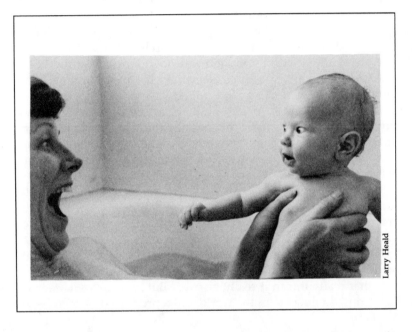

Larry Heald

I felt the urge to push at 10:00 a.m.; I needed to lie back propped up by pillows and really concentrate on my breathing to stay on top of the sensations of discomfort. A half hour later Lorraine said it was time for my mom and the kids to come in to see the baby being born. I remember thinking, No, not yet—it can't be coming this soon! I was blowing hard, trying not to push because there was a stinging sensation, and I didn't want to tear. Lorraine was massaging me with olive oil, which helped. Kate had just arrived. I was really glad that she was able to be there—and just in time!

It was hard pushing the baby out, and I would stop pushing in mid-contraction and blow so as not to tear. Lorraine continued to stretch and massage my perineum as I pushed. At 10:50 a.m., Jacob Campbell Shafer was born. When his head came through, I started laughing, it felt so good. Pushing his shoulders out was pretty hard, and I knew he was considerably bigger than my two girls had been. When he came out, Ramona said, "It's a boy!" He was beautiful. My dad came in to watch Eric cut the umbilical cord. It was wonderful seeing the baby lying on my belly turning pink. Lorraine weighed him at eight and a half pounds with a blanket around him. Eric and the girls took him to give him a Leboyer bath.

I asked for some privacy with Kate and Lorraine so I could concentrate on delivering the placenta. I didn't feel any more contractions, but they helped me up to a squatting position, and I easily pushed the placenta out. What a relief that was, mentally and physically. I felt that my job was now done. I realized that I had been more anxious about delivering the placenta than I had thought.

Eric brought Jacob to me, and he nursed right away. I was surprised at the intensity of the uterine contractions after the birth. These were more uncomfortable than some of my labor contractions and especially painful during nursing. Deep breathing helped.

Jacob's birth was one of the best experiences of my life. With each of my children, the birth was more wonderful than the birth before. Everything happened exactly as I had hoped. My mother said it was the most beautiful thing she had ever seen in her life. I remember seeing tears in my father's eyes and feeling the warmth of my family all around me. What a magic moment! I kept thinking, Was that really it, can it really be over? But, of course, it was just beginning—a new life in the world and a precious new member of our family.

*A note from Eric:* I only wish to add how much credit I give Vicky for maintaining a strong, healthy body and spirit. It was a miracle beyond description for me to directly experience my wife giving natural childbirth. Women cannot be given too much respect for performing such a wonderful act.

*Victoria, a graduate of Sonoma State University, lives on a rural homestead with her husband and three children. As well as having been a foster parent for eight years, she has continued her studies in early childhood education. She and her husband built and operate a state-licensed preschool on their homestead. Among her other interests are organic gardening and raising farm animals.*

# A Breech Delivery

by Nora Sain

The story of my daughter's birth is short, especially when compared to the hubbub of preparation. She was lying breech from the time anyone was willing to say. That ruled out a homebirth as an option in the minds of my birth attendants. I did visualizations and pelvic tilts, and submitted to several tries at external version, but it seemed the baby was firm in its choice of position.

I visited the nearest specialist reputed to let women try a vaginal birth for a breech delivery rather than doing a routine cesarean section. I knew I would be able to do whatever was necessary for the baby's birth, but I had not adequately steeled myself for the disempowering attitude of the doctor. I reacted with near silence throughout the exam and found tears silently flooding over as I peered through the window of the delivery room. Fortunately, my husband and I had reviewed my concerns the evening before, and he was able to step in as my spokesperson. It took the perceptiveness of my midwife at the Clinic to remind me that I was the one having the baby, for which I will always be grateful.

By the time my due date was two days away, I was quite accustomed to frequent Braxton-Hicks contractions. I was merely noticing the contractions as I walked across town to the house where we were staying, but I was aware that a couple of them stopped my walking.

Shortly after I arrived home, my husband and I went to bed and he was soon asleep. I, however, was wide awake. I lay on one side and then the other, on my back, and even on my stomach. Finally I poked my husband and said, "You know, I think they're beginning to hurt." He rolled over. I got up and found I was much more comfortable walking around. So I walked around for a while, and then I walked around and around for a while. And that's how I spent my labor. My absence eventually penetrated my husband's sleep, and he got up and walked around with me—around and around the living room. The most intense period for me was during an attempt to stop walking and rest so I wouldn't wear out. I remember thinking, Well, this is no picnic!

Since it was my first baby we figured we had plenty of time and

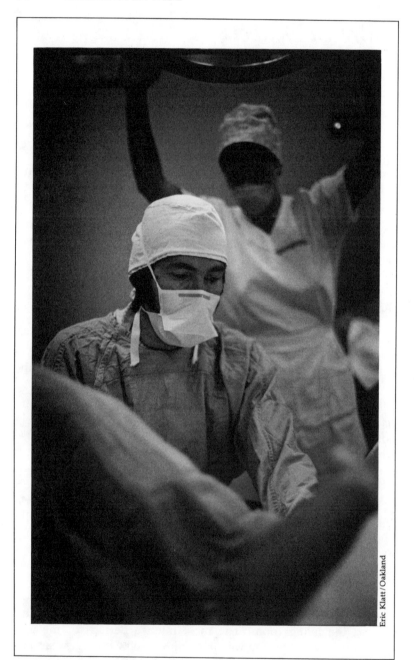

Eric Klatt/Oakland

would wait until dawn to pack for the forty-five minute drive to the hospital. I worked the bathroom into my rounds for periodic runs or dry heaves. It was during one of these pauses that I noticed the bloody show and felt the urge to push—it was unmistakable. We were astounded.

All our carefully made plans! My husband frantically called around to make new arrangements while I got it in my head to take a shower. It was all we could do to get to the local hospital where the bleary-eyed staff graciously accommodated us. They settled me into a room, only to have to move me to the delivery room. It felt very strange to be moved with "something" between my legs. We weren't able to go straight to the delivery room because someone else was using it. The bag of waters broke in the doctor's attempt to determine my dilation.

The pushing came next. I no longer felt an intense urge to push, and I didn't have a sense of how effective my pushes were; I simply followed instructions. I had read that the uterus often didn't need conscious help, so I didn't worry about it. At this point I remembered my carefully rehearsed breathing, but it seemed irrelevant. I guess the staff was scurrying around preparing everything, but I was oblivious.

A couple more pushes and she was almost out. There was an intense moment when her forehead got hung up, but the doctor nipped a small episiotomy, and she was out. A few suctions of mucus cleared her throat, and I finally got to hold her and feel her against me. The doctor and staff removed the placenta and stitched the episiotomy while we goo-gooed at our new family member. We welcomed our daughter and the new day at the same time.

*Nora moved to the country with her husband after they both completed graduate level education. Their homestead dreams have settled into a manageable garden, chickens and an essentially finished owner-built home which is powered by alternative energy. They spend much of their time in community-related activities. Their daughter is growing, vibrant and curious, a reminder to them of the mystery and miracle of life. Nora gave birth to a second daughter four years after her first. The baby died of a rare infection that the most sophisticated medical technology could not control. Nora says, "My life continues in greater touch with reality than before."*

# A Dream Come True

by Pat Weaver

It was September 1, Labor Day. I awoke at 4:00 a.m. —my bag of water had broken. Waves of excitement filled my body. I'm going to have my baby today, I thought. I quickly shook my husband, Peter, and told him the news. Half asleep, he asked if I was having any contractions. I paused a second, then answered, "No, I don't think so."

Peter then explained, "Remember what the midwives said. If you're not having any contractions, try and get more sleep."

Try and get more sleep, I thought. How can you tell a woman who's been waiting nine months for her baby to get more sleep?

I got up and went downstairs. I still needed to sterilize the sheets for the birth. I walked around the house doing my Lamaze breathing and prebirth chores. The more I walked, the closer the contractions seemed to come. They were still very mild even though they were coming at three-minute intervals.

"Peter," I yelled, "you'd better get Kathleen." She was to be our midwife. I had grown very close to her while attending the prenatal yoga classes at the Clinic. In class, Kathleen helped us visualize the birth of our babies. This visualization inspired me to design the baby's birth announcement with an open lotus flower spilling bright stars.

It was 5:30 a.m. when Peter sprang out of bed. I asked him to build a fire in our woodstove before he left. After a few gulps of coffee, he was off to get Kathleen.

It was 7:30 a.m. when he finally arrived with Kathleen and her four-year-old son Joaquin; he had had trouble finding her. "I'm so happy to see you," I exclaimed, as we gave each other a big hug. She then told me why Joaquin was with her. She had promised him he could come to the next birth she attended, although she hadn't expected it to be mine (it was nine days before my due date).

Kathleen sat on the floor next to my chair timing my contractions, which were now two minutes apart but still manageable. She then phoned Kate, our backup midwife, and my friend Suzelle, who was to take pictures of the birth (it had only been a month since I had taken pictures at her delivery), and they both arrived shortly.

The bed and birth supplies were set up in our living room. I was feeling hungry and asked for some tea and toast. I lay down on the bed but had a hard time finding a comfortable position. The tea and toast I had just eaten started to upset my stomach. I felt like I needed to vomit but was too lazy to get up, so Kate and Kathleen walked me to the bathroom. I threw up and felt much better. My contractions were getting stronger.

I lay back on the bed and tried again to find a comfortable position. I was restless. I wanted to be close to Peter. His body was warm and made me feel relaxed and secure, yet I didn't want to burden him for any length of time with my weight. Our house was also getting extremely hot; the fire Peter had made early in the morning was now combining with an outdoor temperature of 80°.

Kathleen suggested I straddle a chair. In this position I could be close to Peter and the midwives, but the chair would hold my weight. With pillows stuffed between the chair and my bottom and belly, I was finally comfortable. Kathleen and Peter sat on chairs facing me, each holding one of my hands. I now started to concentrate on settling my mind and body. Through each contraction I would perform a series of long, deep breaths, exhaling with a low sound. The contraction and the breathing became my focus.

I sat in this position for three hours with occasional trips to the bed so my dilation could be checked. Joaquin would appear at this time for a quick listen to the baby's heartbeat on the fetoscope. There were times in my laboring hours when the contractions would start to pull me away from my focus. The midwives would immediately tune in and pull me through with words of encouragement. I felt their love and warmth all around me. I knew I could continue. Lorraine arrived at noon. "I can't think of a better way to spend Labor Day," she said. I felt wonderful having all the midwives with me.

I began to feel the urge to push. Almost fully dilated with only a lip of the cervix to go, I used the Lamaze "blowing" technique for the next few contractions. Then, I was fully dilated. I was happy to have all those laboring hours over with.

It was time to push. I could feel a contraction coming on so I gulped in a big breath of air. With great effort I flung my head back and used my abdominal muscles to push down. The longer I pushed, the harder it was to hold my breath. Air escaped rapidly from my mouth. I tried to gulp more air but couldn't sustain the force of pushing down, too. The contraction ended and I felt awful. The pushing force was powerful, but I didn't seem to have the right approach to control it and make it work for me. I was confused. "I don't want to push," I stated firmly to the midwives.

"That's all right," they replied, "you can pant through the next contraction." Panting was easy compared to pushing, yet I didn't feel right being so passive when I could be pushing my baby out. Peter then remembered some important information we had learned in our Lamaze class. During my first pushing contraction, I had arched my back. The correct pushing position is leaning forward. Kathleen then suggested a way to help me hold my breath longer. With all this new and useful information, I was eager to try pushing again.

A contraction was starting. "Slow, deep breath in," the midwives reminded me. "Curl over, push, hold it, a little longer. Push! Push! Good work." Ahhh! I did it! "Relax, lie back," the midwives said. Kate and Peter quickly checked my body for tension I might still be holding. A new contraction was starting and I eagerly met it with strength and determination. With each pushing effort I made low, grunting noises. I'm sure these primal sounds would seem strange to anyone who has never been through labor.

By 1:30 p.m. we could see the top of the baby's head. "The baby has hair," Kathleen told me. She held a mirror so I could see the curly black locks of hair protruding from the birth canal.

Now it was time to stop pushing and start blowing. A contraction was coming. Peter firmly placed his hands on my belly. Lorraine's eyes met mine as she led me through the breathing. The baby's head was crowning and forcing my skin to stretch quickly, causing a burning sensation that was hard to bear. Kathleen slowly worked to ease the head out.

The midwives helped Peter and me position our hands to catch the baby. Suzelle moved about trying to find the perfect camera angle. With the next contraction the head was out. Kathleen and Kate worked quickly to suction the baby's nose. Our hands were firmly placed around the baby's head. No one spoke. With one more contraction the baby was out and being lifted onto my belly. It all happened so quickly. One moment there was only a lump under my skin and the next moment we were staring into the eyes of a newly born being.

"What a beautiful baby!" I cried. I couldn't help but say this over and over.

Soon I realized I didn't even know the baby's sex. I looked and mistook the umbilical cord for a penis. "Is it a boy?" I asked.

With a laugh Lorraine replied, "Of course not!" She and Kath-

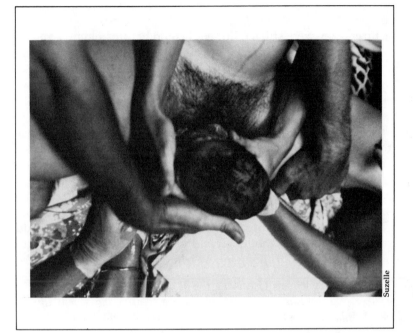

Suzelle

leen both knew I had proclaimed this baby to be a girl throughout my pregnancy.

"She has a name," I said as my eyes focused on Peter. "It's Acacia."

When I first came to California with Peter, I fell in love with the acacia trees that were in bloom at the time. The cotton-puff flowers could be smelled for miles. The acacia tree has always brought to my mind fond memories of my first impressions of California and the love Peter and I shared.

Acacia lay contentedly on my belly. I moved her to my breast and she eagerly started to suck. The midwives gathered together. We were all smiles and Suzelle took our picture. It seemed so natural to be in our home with our friends and our newborn baby. With the midwives' help, our dream of a homebirth had come true.

🐞　　🐞　　🐞

*A note from Peter:* Our delivery experience was full of surprises for me. Though I began the morning exhausted, I found I was continually picking up energy from the others: the midwives, Pat and Acacia herself. The vernix was a surprise too. Nobody told me babies come lanolin-coated. It looked so strangely white against her purple skin. When I wiped it off my hands to take some pictures, they were still so slippery I could hardly hold my camera. But the most astonishing aspect of our delivery was that a child could enter the world so placidly—not screaming, choking or even crying. I had always thought it was a huge trauma. I'm sure we were lucky to have such a perfect delivery.

During the final pushes, as Kathleen did a perineal massage with olive oil to help Pat's skin stretch over Acacia's head, a phrase from my childhood came back to me: "Thou anointest my head with oil." Three other quotations from the Twenty-third Psalm began to take on meaning as symbols for birth, everybody's first brush with death: "My cup runneth over," "The Valley of the Shadow of Death," and "Dwell in the House of the Lord." For one who had not practiced organized religion in a long time, it was odd for me to have these thoughts, and yet appropriate to the miraculous experience of bringing a new being into the light of day.

*Pat moved to Northern California ten years ago from Chicago. She is a member of a local dance group and teaches creative movement to preschool children. She lives with her husband and daughter and is expecting her second child.*

# A Father's Story

by Peter Stern

It's 1:00 a.m.: Janet gets up to go to the bathroom and ends up with a puddle of water on the floor. It takes me a few seconds to realize that it's her waters breaking and not just an accident. And what are these pains she's feeling every three minutes? Seems like labor, ten days early. But we're ready, having just gone to the city last weekend to buy the rest of the essentials (diapers, pails, etc.) that we didn't get at the two showers the week before.

These contractions are intense, irregularly spaced, lasting twenty to thirty seconds and making Janet uncomfortable enough that she has to breathe through them. I figure this is early labor, and it will be sporadic throughout the day and not really get going until later in the afternoon. So, we should just try to get some sleep. Janet figures it's going to go quickly and is slightly apprehensive about it happening too fast. I, of course, don't have any sterile gloves to check dilation, having thought I'd have plenty of time to bring them home from the Clinic. At any rate, it's definitely happening.

The first two hours go by quickly—there's no going back to sleep even if we wanted to. I remember ground rule number one about early labor: Don't get too excited all at once, just let it happen. Sure! My heart's pounding from the beginning. Oh boy, it's happening, we're going to meet our baby real soon. But it's the Fourth of July, how damn patriotic can you get!

3:00 a.m.: Contractions are still intense, still at irregular intervals and irregular duration. We call Kathleen and let her know. She sounds excited and decides to come out with some supplies. I breathe through contractions with Janet. Kathleen arrives, and I do a dilation check: only 1 centimeter and the head is still fairly high. Kathleen suggests that Janet and I stay in bed, caress, smooch and let things progress—she's going home and will come back later in the morning.

Janet's slightly discouraged, having thought it would be moving faster. We go back to bed, I give her a massage and we breathe through contractions while half asleep. Time starts passing more slowly, and I try to stay awake. Janet gets up and paces through

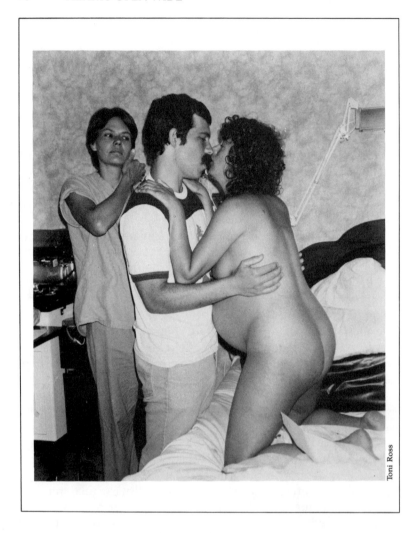

Toni Ross

the contractions and gets things together for the hospital.

7:30 a.m.: I do another dilation check and it's 3 centimeters. It's hard trying not to get too excited, too anxious, thinking it could go real fast from here on but knowing it's probably going to be a long day. Janet wants to go in to the hospital, and this sounds like a good idea. I've been a little put off at the idea of a hospital birth, but at the birthing room it seems as if we'll have control over how it goes, and Janet will feel secure in having the hospital backup.

We take a long slow drive to town. Janet labors in the back of the station wagon. It's a beautiful morning although it feels like it's going to be a scorcher. When we get to the hospital we go straight to the birthing room, and contrary to my fears of hospital intervention, we're virtually left alone. I call Kathleen, Kate and our friend Toni. Dr. Bill is at the nurses' station, and is surprised to see me and to find out that Janet is in labor. It doesn't feel weird to be at the hospital—it's like being around family.

10:00 a.m.: Kate comes in. Janet and I (mostly Janet) are working hard getting through contractions, trying to stay loose and thinking, Open, let the contractions do their work of opening the cervix. Janet's doing well at breathing, relaxing, concentrating on staying in the here and now. I knew she would although she had been uncertain of her ability to stay with it and not act like a baby.

Kate does a dilation check: 6 centimeters. All right! Things are progressing steadily—slowly but steadily. At this rate we'll have a baby before too long. Kathleen comes in, followed by Toni. Throughout the morning we are all with a common cause—getting a baby born. It feels good. Janet, on the other hand, has more pressing matters to think about, i.e., getting through the next contraction. She's had to change breathing patterns to a "pant-pant-blow" cycle and change positions. We're breathing together, keeping eye contact, staying right here. I'm getting slightly hyperventilated, but it's worth it. Janet is beautiful to watch during contractions—totally concentrating, rocking back and forth almost catlike in her movements. When she's blowing out, she reminds me of the pictures of the face of the wind that I've seen on maps.

2:00 p.m.: The contractions are very intense. Janet is now groaning through them. Kathleen says she's changed from cat-mode into tiger-mode. Kate does a check and feels an anterior cervical lip. We work with some position changes and get Janet to push during contractions. The midwives are great as pushing coaches: Down and outward, open, legs relaxed, rest and breathe between contractions.

Pushing turns out to be the hardest work yet. It hurts, and she doesn't even feel a real urge to push. This baby has a big head and that, coupled with an anterior lip, slows things down. It's discouraging. We thought that as soon as we got through transition we would be home free—a few pushes and out would pop a baby. But Janet's been pushing one hour, two hours, and things are moving so slowly. Little thoughts keep creeping into my head:

Cephalo-pelvic disproportion, swollen anterior cervical lip—are we going to wind up with a c-section? Where's the baby already? I'm exhausted, Janet's exhausted. She's been pushing with all her might every two to four minutes now for two hours. But there's nothing else to do but stay with it, bear down and push the baby out.

The swollen lip remains a problem. Kate manually reduces it a couple of times, and the head does seem to be moving downward and outward, if ever so slowly. Janet's really doing great, working hard, staying so focused, so concentrated, never once losing it. We try a new position—on her right side, semi-reclining with her left knee to her chest. This seems to help; the pushes are now getting somewhere. Janet can feel the head with her fingers, which is encouraging. Soon we can see some hair. I breathe a few sighs of relief knowing that soon this little one will be born.

5:00 p.m.: The head, a hairy one at that, is now crowning and pushing open the perineum. It's truly a big head, and it's taking its time stretching things out. It gets to a point where Janet's perineum doesn't look like it can stretch any further. Kate makes a small cut, and the head emerges in a few more pushes. A cute, scrunched-up purple face looks out at us. Another push and the shoulders, trunk and legs slither out.

5:19 p.m.: A boy! He's put onto Janet's belly where he promptly evacuates the contents of his rectum, as if to welcome himself to the outside world; but who cares, he's out, he's breathing, and he's pinked up. He does have an incredibly molded head, a huge caput, but he's beautiful anyhow.

The feelings are hard to put into words—joy, thankfulness, love, euphoria—definitely euphoria, an exhausted euphoria. Now we can relax, lie back and spend some time with this little guy whom we've been waiting so long to meet. He quickly gets into sucking and just as quickly falls asleep. Janet's been incredible throughout the entire process. I am in awe of her ability to have been so focused, relaxed and beautiful at the same time, and I feel very lucky that we're together.

*Peter, a naturopathic physician, graduated from the National College of Naturopathic Medicine in Portland, Oregon in 1981 and now practices at the Clinic. He spent four months in Beijing, China studying traditional Chinese medicine and attended the San Francisco College of Acupuncture and Oriental Medicine.*

# On the Road Again

by Joanne Grace

---

It started just like any other day. Ho hum, when's this little child coming? I was three weeks late according to the dates. I had finally resigned myself to being forever pregnant, although I knew better. Then I started getting little tickles way down low—maybe, just maybe! I didn't want to get our hopes up, but I told Chan that I was feeling *something*. I couldn't help thinking that it would be soon.

Becca, our neighbor and midwife, came to invite us to a birthday party that day. We could meet our other neighbors, have some fun and pass the time. We walked over to the party and spent the day eating birthday cake and playing games. I was rushing but wouldn't admit it was happening. I'd start to rush, and it would come on strong until my face would flush, and then it would fade. I felt juicy and warm—inside-out. The women at the party tuned into the energy and gave us lots of love and space. I was tiring out and decided to go home and rest up for the birth. So, up the hill and into bed.

Just when I was really relaxed and everyone else was asleep, the rushes came. Boy, did they come! Real contractions, no denying it. We're having a baby. I woke Chan and Ryan, my three-year-old son. We crammed the VW Bug with blankets, birth supplies and our dog. Since we were living far from town, we had decided to have our little one at Kathleen's house where we would feel more secure.

Down the road we went, stopping to pee and to lock and unlock gates. We stopped at Becca's to tell her we were on our way to Kathleen's. She said she'd grab a sandwich and be right behind us. (If only we'd known!) Back down the road, still peeing and opening gates. Chan stopped the car for every contraction to help me integrate the energy which was so intense it was coming out my mouth: low, loud exhalations. I wished the contractions would stop until we got to Kathleen's, but knew that was absurd. I could visualize my cervix opening, opening with every rush. I guess if I'd had a minute to think about it, I would have realized that I was in transition. My legs were shaking and every rush was more powerful than the last, and they were coming closer together. Our focus was on getting to Kathleen's, twenty-five miles down the road, and we'd hardly traveled five. Time and space were unreal. I just wanted to get out of the car. *Where is Becca anyway?*

The rushes were strong and fast, still coming out my mouth, the only thing I could do. Ryan was worried about me, but Chan reassured him that our baby was coming. He understood. It was obvious that we wouldn't make it to Kathleen's, but we didn't know what we should do: stop or go? I felt my cervix complete dilation: 7, 8, 9, 10 centimeters! Then I felt the head move down the birth canal. I could remove myself from my body and feel my uterus contract and push the baby out. "Well, Chan, we're not going to make it."

We pulled to the side of the road. It was dark—no flashlight, no moon. I was having one continuous contraction. Chan pulled my pants off (you can guess where my brains were, pushing out my little one while I still had my pants on!) and felt between my legs and said, "Yep, it's a baby." With that, the water bag ballooned out of me and just as easy as pie the head slid into it. All I knew was that I couldn't see anything, and I couldn't hear my babe. Chan tore the bag from our baby's head and pulled it away from the nose and mouth. (How he could see what was going on, I don't know. He later called it "cosmic vision.") There still was no sound. He felt for the cord, it was around the neck. He pulled to loosen it and out came the body. I lifted my sweater and put the baby on my body to keep it warm. *Where is Becca?* Chan got the birth pack and found a soft blanket at the bottom to wrap the baby in—sterile stuff all over the place. I wondered, Is it a boy or a girl? I thought it was a boy because I felt the cord between the legs and assumed it was a penis. But Chan investigated further and discovered a girl. A girl! Our daughter! *Whatever happened to Becca?*

After some time (time and space were still unreal) and more contractions, out came the placenta. Chan caught it in the tub we had intended to use for the Leboyer bath. Oh well! We clamped the cord with the clips the midwives had given us "just in case." Ryan found a knife for Chan, who cut the cord. All the sterile stuff went into the trunk and we continued on to Kathleen's.

We met Becca and Mary on their search for us. They were amazed and happy to find us with our healthy baby girl. Becca had called Mary and went a back way to pick her up. She thought she'd meet us at Kathleen's. But, when they arrived and found that we weren't there, they knew what had happened. They followed us

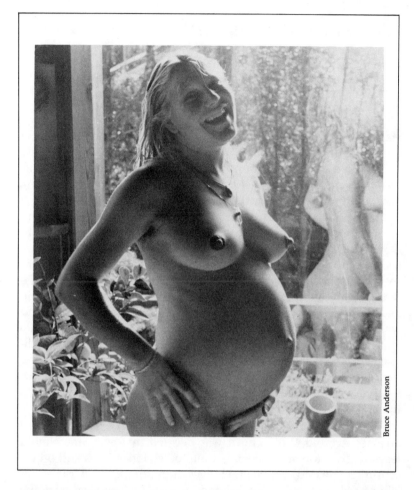

Bruce Anderson

back to Kathleen's. They checked the baby and me and all was well. No rips. She weighed seven and a half pounds.

Amber Meraki, perfect woman child, Gypsy baby. She was conceived while we were traveling, born on the road. The moon was Void of Course, and she was born in the caul. She is a special person indeed. Her light shines on all who see her. Welcome, little soul, drop of light.

*As part of her studies as an aspiring lay midwife, Joanne has completed the Doula Training Program at the Clinic and assists the midwives at births. She lives with her partner and their children on a communal homestead. She is a beadwork artist and enjoys reggae music.*

# Our Anniversary Gift

by Melinda Stahl

It was the day after my thirty-second birthday, and my due date was a week away. As we drove the last four miles of dirt road on the way home from a day at the county fair, I felt the first mild contractions. Ron and I went to bed that night wondering if this was the start of my labor. I only slept four or five hours, waking now and then to a contraction.

The next day I continued to have mild contractions. Some were ten to fifteen minutes apart, but there was no regular pattern to them, and I took a long walk to visit a neighbor. That night they became stronger, and I couldn't sleep. I was planning a homebirth, so around 1:00 a.m. Ron tried to reach our midwife on the CB radio. Fortunately, another lady overheard Ron's call on her radio and as they were talking, Lorraine heard her name mentioned and woke up. She got her partner, Kathleen, and they arrived at 3:00 a.m. My cervix was completely effaced but only 1 centimeter dilated. After a few hours of talking with the midwives and receiving their love, support and reassurance, we all tried to get some sleep. I only slept a couple of hours and woke to some intense contractions.

In the morning several friends whom I'd asked to be at the birth arrived. Around 11:00 a.m. it was decided that everyone should leave to give Ron and me some time to be alone. I was still only 1 centimeter dilated, and the midwives didn't think I'd go into active labor until later in the day. I already felt uncomfortable during the contractions, but I had no idea how much more painful they would get. Working as an RN for ten years, I had seen many women in labor; therefore, I knew it wasn't easy and that the term "labor" is an accurate one. But I had been so at peace, happy and joyful during my pregnancy and had prayed so often to our beloved Lord, that I really expected I would have a quick labor. Well, so much for expectations! One of my midwives had told me not to have any, but I obviously hadn't listened.

An hour after everyone left, my contractions became more intense and more frequent. I was trying to do the slow deep breathing recommended by the Bradley method. As the afternoon slowly passed by, the pain became so intense that sometimes the breathing turned into crying. I took a shower, we tried to make love, we tried to take a walk, but it was just too hard. I tried gripping a comb in my hands*, but that didn't seem to help either. Although we were both so tired from lack of sleep, it amazed us to find that we could actually fall asleep for the three or four minutes between contractions.

Ron kept trying to get Lorraine on the CB, but reception was poor and we were unable to reach anyone. Around 5:00 p.m. my brother and his girlfriend drove to town and called Lorraine to tell her I was having a hard time, but for some reason I didn't specifically tell them to ask her to come back as soon as she could.

The contractions were regular and so intense that I felt I must be dilating. But when I checked myself (I had done vaginal exams at work), I was disappointed and depressed to find my cervix still only 1 centimeter dilated. I kept visualizing my cervix opening and chanted, "Open, open." I have given a drug called Nisentil to women in labor and have seen how much it can help to relax and relieve pain without stopping labor. I was hurting and was so tired that I didn't care any more about having a natural homebirth. I just wanted something to relieve the pain. I also thought that maybe something was wrong because I wasn't dilating. I kept waiting to hear a car drive up, hoping it would be Lorraine and Kathleen. I really needed their reassurance and support. Ron was just as dismayed as I was. This was his first experience with birth, and he had wanted a hospital birth all along, while I'd insisted on having it at home.

Around 7:00 p.m., Bobby and Robin came back from town, and when I heard the car and then realized it wasn't Lorraine and Kathleen, I burst into tears. At that point I decided to go to the hospital; all I could think about was a shot of Nisentil. I was still doing the slow deep breathing. It hadn't occurred to either of us to change my breathing pattern although we'd practiced the panting and blowing in our prenatal class just a few weeks earlier.

Ron finally reached Lorraine on the CB. They were just leaving to come back. Ron told her I had decided to go to the hospital. She

---

*A reflexology technique which is said to stimulate points on the hand directly related to the uterus and to facilitate smooth, rapid and relatively painless functioning of the uterus.

asked to talk to me, and after making sure that this was really what I wanted to do, she said she'd call the doctor and meet us there. After seven hours of intense pain without dilation, I was tired and discouraged, and the decision to do something made me feel better.

Arriving at the small rural hospital where I'd worked for six years, I was greeted by friends and fellow workers who helped me

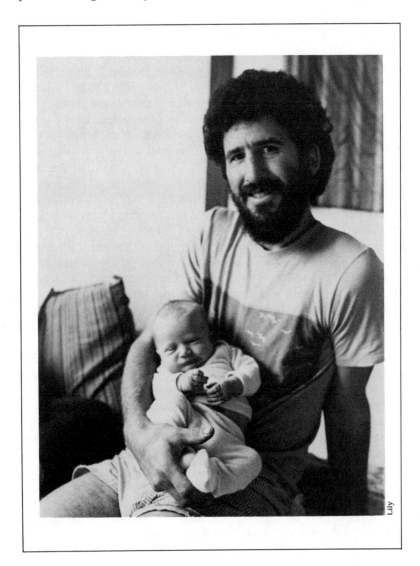

to the bed in the alternative birth room. I always knew that if I ended up at the hospital, this option was available. The midwives arrived shortly after we did, and they immediately had me start panting and blowing instead of the slow deep breathing (and crying) I had been doing. It was amazing how much better I felt after this change, and with their support, I didn't need to take the Nisentil. Mark, the doctor on call that night, did a vaginal exam, and I was 5 centimeters dilated. He figured the bouncy ride down our hill helped to dilate me. Now why didn't I take a ride earlier!

I was feeling so much better, I wanted to go home (me, irrational?). After talking it over with everyone, Ron and I decided that we should stay. Dr. Mark was very understanding and held off admitting me until we'd made our decision. It was around 8:00 p.m. by then.

After what seemed like eons but was really only four to five hours, I was completely dilated, though there was still a cervical lip. Dr. Mark finally broke my bag of waters and helped the head come past the lip. Then started the long, hard stage of pushing. I've never worked so hard in my life. Mark did some perineal massage. He said there was a good chance I would tear, so I asked him to do an episiotomy. I just wanted it over with, I was so tired and needed to rest. Finally, at 3:17 a.m., our daughter was born, healthy and beautiful. She was quite blue at first but started to pink up as they gave her a little oxygen, and I cuddled her in my arms. After fifty hours of mild labor and fifteen hours of hard labor, she was finally here. It was our sixth wedding anniversary—what a present we got, what a day we had!

But it wasn't quite over. While Ron and the nurse took Veronica and put her in the Leboyer bath, I tried to push out the placenta. It wouldn't come, so Mark stitched me up and then I tried again to expel it. As I pushed, Mark gently pulled, and the cord came off in his hand! He had to remove the stitches and manually remove the placenta. Fortunately, he was able to do this in the alternative birth room while I did some heavy deep breathing. The usual procedure is to take the mother to surgery and anesthetize her. It was quite painful, but after all I'd been through, I certainly didn't want to have to go to surgery too.

Over the years I've come to believe that everything happens for a reason. Although I'd planned a homebirth, it turned out to be a good thing that we were in the hospital. Lorraine was glad we were there because, although she'd done several manual removals of the placenta, she didn't feel comfortable with them. Then, around 2:00 a.m., Lorraine received a phone call and had to coach a husband and wife who were having a precipitate birth at home.** Lorraine and Kathleen were the only midwives available that weekend, and if they had been at our home, they couldn't have been reached by phone. Another woman came to the hospital that night and Lorraine went right from my birth to be with her. So it turned out best for everyone that we had gone to the hospital.

We were discharged around noon the next day. Though weak and exhausted, we rejoiced that the good Lord had blessed us with His gift of love. He has blessed us in so very many ways, and we thank Him and praise His name.

---

**See "The Telephone Baby," p. 226.

*Before the birth of her daughter Veronica, Melinda worked at the local eighteen-bed hospital. After returning to work, she discovered that she was pregnant once again. Her dream of a homebirth was finally fulfilled when, to everyone's surprise, she delivered a set of twins. Ron is a self-employed carpenter and takes an active part in the care of his children. Melinda loves gardening, reading, exercising and spiritual work.*

# Just in Time

by Susan Vaughn

---

As I lay in bed that first night, I listened to four separate breaths in our family bed. Mine was hoarse and ragged after the harsh breathing of second stage labor. My son Nathan, two and a half years old, was still making the sucking sounds he had made since he was born, even though he stopped nursing seven months before when I found I was pregnant again. My husband's breathing was deep and even, as usual. My newborn baby girl lay beside me. Her breathing was irregular, as a newborn's always is. I lay there and thought, Six hours ago I was pregnant and in the most intense part of labor, trying to push the baby out. Now I'm lying peacefully in bed enjoying the complete absence of pain, and everyone I love is within arm's reach of me.

Labor, that long-awaited, much-desired but also feared end of pregnancy, had become only a memory. Our lives had made yet another turn. None of us lying in bed that night would ever be the same. What had changed? A baby had been born that day.

❧        ❧        ❧

My labor began at 1:00 a.m. I awoke feeling a painful contraction and the need to go to the bathroom. I went back to bed and slept until nearly 6:00 a.m. My contractions were seven to ten minutes apart and irregular, so I wasn't convinced I was in labor. I had always thought that labor contractions, unlike Braxton-Hicks, were supposed to happen at regular intervals and gradually come closer together. Mine didn't seem to be doing that.

Being a school teacher, I had certain responsibilities to fulfill that day before I could have my baby: Write lesson plans, contact the principal and get in touch with the substitute teacher. I went to school to put everything in order. My contractions were so far apart and irregular I felt embarrassed alerting everyone and saying, "I might be in labor." I even thought there was a chance I'd be back at work the next day with a baby still in my belly.

When I got home, my husband and son were eating breakfast. I informed Tom of my progress and told him how skeptical I was. It was 10:00 a.m. and I wondered whether I should call my midwives, but there didn't seem to be any hurry. We went for a walk and my contractions suddenly became more frequent, although they were still irregular. By the time we got home, they were three to four minutes apart, but once I sat down and rested they went right back to seven minutes apart.

I was thoroughly confused. The contractions were beginning to really hurt, which confused me even more. I finally called Kate at 11:00 a.m. I explained my situation to her and from my description, she said it sounded like I was still in early labor. Since she was working at the Clinic, she didn't want to leave until she had to, which suited me fine. Next I called Lorraine and she said pretty much the same thing. She would come to my house within the next two hours to check my progress. If I was still in early labor, she would go back home. This relieved me tremendously since I knew in my heart that I wanted to labor alone without anyone monitoring me.

After I called the midwives, we had lunch and I sat on the porch feeling the contractions come and go. They hurt but they were still seven minutes apart, and I wasn't particularly concerned about them. At 12:30 p.m., Tom put Nathan to bed for his nap. That was when things really began to happen, and I knew beyond the shadow of a doubt that I was, indeed, in labor.

My contractions sped up dramatically. Tom timed them; they were two and a half minutes apart, lasting a minute and a half. I hardly knew when one ended and another began. I started pacing the floor, back and forth, back and forth, holding my belly and ordering Tom around as if he were one of my kids at school. I ordered him into the kitchen to wash the lunch dishes. Then, almost immediately, I ordered him to the phone to call the midwives. When we finally contacted Kate, I tried to explain the situation as accurately as I could. Contractions were close together and painful. But, "No, I'm not using any special breathing techniques with them."

Kate asked, "Are you feeling pushy?"

"No," I said, but I suspected I would be feeling that way very soon. I felt confused and was having trouble communicating. These are both symptoms of transition, but at the time I didn't recognize them.

About ten minutes after I hung up (more pacing, more ordering, more complaining—"My God, I'm going to have to do this all day"), I had a bloody show. The contractions were coming very fast. I ordered Tom back to the phone, but when the Clinic answered we were told that Kate was on her way.

I went back to my pacing, and Tom went back to the dishes. It occurred to me that I was going to have a baby very soon and that I had done nothing but yell at Tom for the past half hour. Pictures flashed through my mind from accounts I had read of husbands and wives working together intensely during labor—husbands lovingly sponging off their laboring wives' foreheads or massaging their backs and breathing through contractions with them. There I was, frantically pacing back and forth, ordering Tom to wash the dishes and make phone calls, complaining all the time. Suddenly the whole situation struck me as hilariously funny. Anyone looking on would think we had a very unsatisfactory relationship, which isn't true at all. I was glad no midwives were there to watch me behaving in this way. Perhaps that is why I wanted to labor alone. If anyone besides Tom had been there, I would have been self-conscious and inhibited, and perhaps labor wouldn't have progressed so quickly.

At this point I was also beginning to get very nervous and more than a little scared. Minutes after my bloody show I began to feel the urge to push. As Tom finished the dishes, I told him I felt like pushing. He told me to breathe. I told him the baby was coming and he'd better get the sterile sheets out. After he started to get them out, I told him to put them away because it wasn't time yet, and they might get dirty. Tom was calmly trying to do everything I asked. I wonder now why he didn't lose his patience with me. He was really wonderful.

Because no midwife was there to check for a cervical lip, I was afraid to start pushing. I breathed through the first pushing contractions pretty well. I was still standing up and didn't know what position I wanted to be in. I couldn't use the bed since my son was still taking a nap. I had learned from my previous midwife that women are less likely to tear in a hands-and-knees position since the head doesn't put as much pressure on the perineum. So I tried that for my next contraction. Actually, I was lying across the couch with my head and chest supported by it, my knees on the floor. To my surprise I found this very comfortable, especially between contractions. I couldn't help but push with my next contraction even though Tom kept saying, "Don't push! Breathe!"

I said, "I can't breathe, I have to push!" I was already "breathing" my lungs out—breathing as deep and fast as I possibly could. Somewhere around this time I said to Tom, "You just can't believe how much this hurts." I just wanted to let him know exactly how I was feeling. I guess I wanted him to appreciate me. (I also look back on this with considerable humor.) The fourth pushing contraction came, and I breathed through it as Tom was commanding me to, but again I couldn't help but push at the end of it. Still no midwives had arrived.

Tom got out the sterile sheets and put them under me. The fifth contraction came, and I knew my baby was crowning. My perineum burned. Tom was massaging me, trying to get me to open up. I told him it hurt. He told me to breathe, and I yelled back that I couldn't and simply screamed through the whole contraction— something I had never done before. My voice sounded strange in my ears, and I hoped I wouldn't wake up Nathan. It was then that my water broke.

The next contraction came with unbelievable force. I opened my mouth and screamed again, and the head was born. I heard nothing from the baby, and my fear rose. There were still no midwives. What if the baby didn't breathe? Tom and the baby were very quiet. Tom told me to keep pushing, and this time I said, "I can't, I don't feel any contractions."

At that moment I heard a car coming up the driveway. It seemed an eternity before Kate and Lorraine walked through the door. The body still had not been born. Lorraine rushed over to support the head and was immediately splattered with a huge burst of blood. Kate discovered that the cord was around the baby's neck. As soon as she removed it, the body slowly slid out. Kalendy Leah began to cry. Her Apgar score was nine, and I had a beautiful, healthy baby. I began to bleed so Kate gave me two shots of Pitocin while Lorraine clamped my uterus with one hand inside my vagina. I put Kalendy to my breast and she nursed right away, which helped to keep my uterus tight. Kate checked me and discovered that I had only one small tear, not even enough to stitch. It was 1:30 p.m., twelve and a half hours after labor had begun.

One hour after Kalendy was born, I felt as good as new. My perineum had stopped burning, and I was no longer in pain and no longer pregnant; my baby was asleep on my chest. Nathan woke up from his nap and sat on his daddy's lap marvelling at the new creature who had come into our household and into our hearts. It was the perfect ending to my long and not-so-perfect pregnancy. I was already beginning to remember, as I had discovered with Nathan, that having a baby is the most incredible high on earth.

❧     ❧     ❧

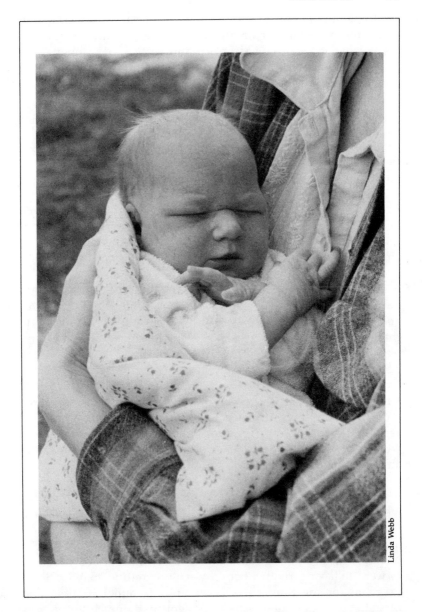

Linda Webb

## ONE LAST TIME

It seems as if I just wrote a birth story—indeed, it has only been fourteen months since Kalendy, my second child, was born. I conceived my third child just four months after Kalendy's birth, but I was not to know this until my first trimester was nearly past. I had no symptoms of pregnancy whatsoever—my energy was high, I had no morning sickness, and since I was nursing, my breasts were not sore and showed no signs of change. These were all the symptoms that had alerted me to my first two pregnancies within days after conceiving.

You can imagine my surprise and denial when my husband began commenting that my usually slim body was taking on the contours of pregnancy. My denial was understandable since I had had two periods after Kalendy's birth, one when she was four months old and the other seven weeks later. It wasn't until other people began asking me if I was pregnant *again* that I myself began to wonder. I had to admit that if I wasn't pregnant, something was wrong. Even I could no longer deny the outward sign of pregnancy—a protruding belly. When I went to the Clinic for a pregnancy test, Kate checked me and sure enough, I was already ten to twelve weeks pregnant. It had only been thirty days since my last period.

Another baby! Not only was I working full time, I was going to have three children under the age of four. What should I do? An abortion seemed to be the best answer, but I knew I couldn't do that. The baby had already been growing for three full months and was a perfectly formed little creature by now—it was soon to become a member of our family.

This pregnancy was a breeze compared to my first two, in which I had spent the first six months throwing up and the last three months feeling uncomfortable with indigestion. My energy level remained unusually high, and for the first time I understood how women could say they felt better during their pregnancies than at any other time in their lives.

Kalendy, who had been a rather fussy and colicky baby, at eight months turned into a sweet, outgoing, uncomplaining little girl who slept all night and was a joy. Nathan, though at times jealous, really loved his sister, and they actually began playing together. All in all, after the first few weeks of emotional anguish had been worked out, everything went smoothly. If I wasn't exactly looking forward to having another baby, I wasn't regretting it either. Being pregnant for the third time, however, was rather routine, and thoughts about the new baby were kept pretty much in the back of my mind.

All this changed as my due date drew closer. I anticipated having another homebirth since my first two children had been born at home. Kate, however, saw things differently. With both

Nathan and Kalendy I had, for some unknown reason, bled profusely after the births. Kate claimed that this put me into a high-risk category; therefore, I should have my baby in the hospital. With each previous birth, my midwife had needed to administer a shot of Pitocin to keep my uterus contracted and to stop the bleeding. Each time this shot was successful, so Kate had a hard time convincing me that it was really necessary to go to the hospital. After all, I thought, the bleeding had stopped and there were no terrible consequences. From my point of view all had gone well. I felt that Kalendy's birth had turned out perfectly; I didn't bleed until my work had been done, and there was a newborn baby lying on my belly. I hardly even noticed the volume of blood Kate claimed was gushing out of my body. Of course, our perspectives were totally different. She walked into the room after my daughter's head was born and immediately had to deal with a highly intense situation that she was responsible for. I simply lay back in euphoria cuddling my infant.

All this discussion of homebirth versus hospital birth brought my pregnancy to a head, and for the first time I really began to think about the birth of my third child. My husband and I were unanimous in our desire not to go to the hospital, but at the same time we knew it would be foolish to try to have the baby by ourselves at home. We also did not want to put Kate in the awkward position of having to come to our house when we knew she didn't want to, even though she had said she would. So, though it depressed me very much, I decided to go to the hospital. I reasoned it would be a novel experience, and Kate had recently gotten hospital privileges, so she could still be my birth attendant.

I soon got accustomed to the idea. And as my pregnancy dragged on to one week, two weeks, three and a half weeks overdue, I think I would have consented to having the baby at Grand Central Station if that would have brought labor on. My due date was a bit uncertain; however, no woman in her ninth month of pregnancy believes her baby would come out one minute later than that long-awaited due date. That you could get any fatter or wait any longer seems impossible.

We discussed going to the hospital for a non-stress test to make sure the baby was all right. In the course of this discussion, we decided that if all systems seemed ready, Kate would go ahead and induce labor. My cervix was already 3 centimeters dilated and 75 percent effaced.

I barely thought about my impending labor all day while I

taught school, except to arrange for babysitters for my two children. I wanted Nathan to participate in this birth, so I arranged to have a friend bring him to the hospital when the birth seemed imminent.

On the way to the hospital we decided on a name for our baby. This was practically the first time we had even seriously discussed it. It seemed strange to think I would be having a baby soon, especially since I was not in labor.

At the hospital I had the non-stress test, and the baby's heart rate was normal, so we decided to go ahead and take the plunge. At 6:00 p.m. Kate broke my water. I immediately went into very light labor with contractons three to five minutes apart but only lasting ten seconds or so. Since it was dinner time, Tom and I went out and we enjoyed a good, peaceful dinner alone without our two children for the first time in months; it occurred to me we would not get another evening out by ourselves for a long time to come.

After eating dinner and then walking around town for an hour, we went back to the hospital to report my progress to Kate. Contractions were still light and short, but I was losing my mucus plug. We sat talking to Kate awhile, but I felt that my labor would progress more quickly if I got up and walked around, so at 9:00 p.m. Tom and I again left the hospital to walk the dark and empty streets of town. This time my contractions seemed to intensify a bit, and I had to stop and breathe through a couple of them. An hour later we were back in the hospital, and this time Kate checked my dilation. I had progressed only one centimeter in four hours. I was now at 4 centimeters dilation—not an encouraging report since I was beginning to feel very tired from my long day's work and my unusual bout of exercise that evening. I decided the best thing I could do was to try to get some sleep. Kate agreed and said if my labor didn't pick up by morning, she would have to give me an IV with Pitocin.

Tom fell asleep almost at once, but, of course, I couldn't get comfortable. To make matters worse, my contractions immediately intensified. Gee, I thought, for 4 centimeters these contractions really hurt! I had to start breathing through them. Seven deep breaths, I counted. Anyone can stand seven deep breaths, I thought. I had to get up to go to the bathroom with each contraction and couldn't sit still. I didn't know what to do with myself. Tom slept on. I was very confused. I sat down to go to the bathroom again, and strangely enough, I felt like pushing. I refused to believe this. It had only been an hour since I was 4 centimeters. I

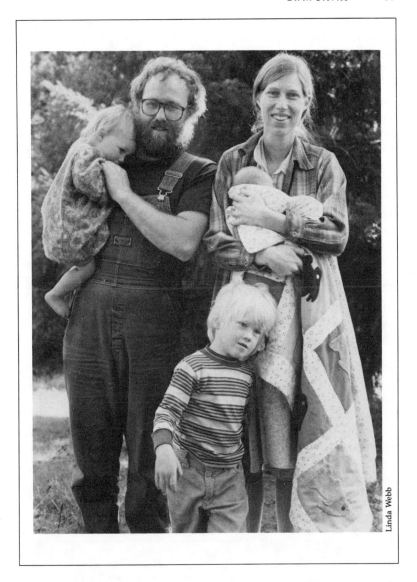

Linda Webb

had another contraction that hurt like hell, and I finally woke Tom. My next contraction was definitely a pushing contraction. I sent Tom on the run to get Kate.

They both rushed into the room. Kate checked me where I stood and told me that I was fully dilated. We piled pillows and a beanbag chair onto the bed. I leaned my head and chest on them in a hands and knees position. Kate was frantically trying to find everything she needed, and suddenly the room filled with strangers and nurses, and everything was happening so fast I couldn't believe it. The pain was intense, and my perineum was on fire. I knew my baby would be born soon, but I just couldn't stand the pain and screamed my heart out. It was 11:27 p.m. and I'm sure I woke the whole hospital, but that scream brought the birth of my new daughter's head. The pain was still intense, but the next contraction birthed the body. Before I knew it, I was lying on my back with Katie Rose in my arms. I couldn't believe it was all over.

My third child was whole and well, and I knew I would never be pregnant again. Within an hour everyone had left the room, and Tom and I were alone in our hospital bed with Katie Rose between us. I felt thankful I didn't have to be in labor all night and was surprised, as always, at the intensity of the experience.

The hospital birth, which I had so feared, turned out to be my easiest and quickest birth. Although it was not the birth I had envisioned, for I was disappointed my son wasn't there, I have good memories of it. Our family had enlarged for the last time, and everyone's place in it had changed once again. Life has been very good to us.

*Susan received her teaching credential from Humboldt State University and pursues her career as the teacher at a one-room rural school. She feels fortunate to be able to combine her job with mothering and gives credit to her husband for his active involvement in the care of their three young children. Her interests include reading, homeopathy, medical self-help, exercise and square dancing.*

# Callie Marie's Birth

by Judy Mirsky

---

Spike and I each have a child from a previous marriage. After marrying, we tried to conceive for two and a half years. We knew our chances were slim, because Spike had had a vasectomy and then a reversal. His doctor told him the operation was successful, but his sperm count was low. When we found out that we were going to have a baby, we decided on a hospital birth with the help and support of a very special midwife.

❧     ❧     ❧

July 7, 4:00 a.m.: My husband Spike left for Sacramento on a business trip. He said he had not slept well thinking that I might go into labor, even though it was still two weeks from my due date. I assured him nothing was going to happen, so he left.

About one hour later, my water broke, waking me up. I had a mild contraction soon afterwards. I left a message for my midwife, Lily, to get in touch with me; then I called another midwife, Becca, and told her what was happening. She said she would stop by our house on her way into town, but it sounded to her like I probably wouldn't have the baby until that night.

Spike called at 8:00 a.m. from 150 miles away just to check on me. For a moment I thought I wouldn't tell him about my water breaking since he planned on being back late that night anyway. But I told him, and he got very excited and said he was coming right back.

By 10:00 a.m. my contractions had gotten stronger, but they were still about forty-five minutes apart. I again tried to reach Lily, without any luck. I left messages everywhere for her.

At 10:45 a.m. Becca and Spike showed up. I was in bed and had had a couple of hard contractions. Becca talked to me for a few minutes and said I still had a long way to go, probably most of the day. She decided not to check me so early to lessen the chance of infection since my water had broken.

Right after Becca left, Spike sat on the bed, and I guess I was so glad to see him that my contractions started getting really strong and coming every five minutes. Spike wanted to call Dr. Bill, but I

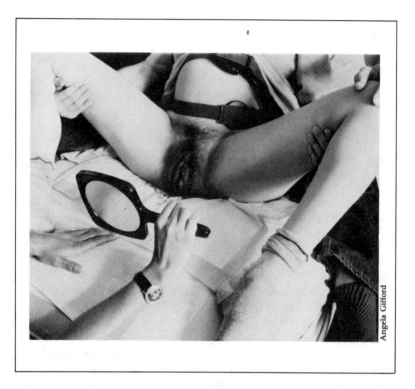

Angela Gifford

was still hoping that Lily would come. Finally, at 12:15 p.m., Spike talked with Bill and told him my contractions were three minutes apart and pretty intense. Bill said to meet him at the hospital at 1:00 p.m. Lily came about five minutes later, and was I glad to see her smiling face! I will always remember her telling me to look into her eyes so she could help me through the contractions. She checked me, and I was 8 centimeters dilated.

She said we'd have to hurry, but the last thing I wanted to do was move. Spike grabbed my suitcase and pillows, and he and Lily helped me into the car. I had one contraction in the car and one in the parking lot of the hospital. The medics rushed out with a wheelchair and wanted me to sit in it, but Lily said, "Not right now, she's having a contraction." After the contraction ended, they pushed me into a waiting room.

Dr. Bill had just gotten there and took Lily's word for it that there was no time to lose. I went right into a semi-private room and was helped onto the bed. Bill asked the nurse if he could set everything up in time, and the nurse said he would try. Dr. Bill then told me that if he couldn't, I would have to go into the delivery room to have my baby.

There wasn't time for anything—Lily was having me blow, I was trying not to push, Bill ran to put on his "greenies." (Everyone else, including me, was still in street clothes.) Dr. Bill and Lily started coaching me—when to blow, pant or push. Spike held on to my hand (or the other way around) and gave me lots of support. The contractions were so intense I didn't think I could go through another one. Lily had me feel the baby's head crowning and held up a little mirror so I could see it. Bill knew I didn't want an episiotomy if I could avoid it, so at that moment he gave me a choice of a little one or one more contraction. I chose the episiotomy, but right then another contraction came, and he said, "We don't need to do one, we've almost got it now." When they said I could finally push, it felt great! I pushed so hard my arms and shoulders were sore for two days. The baby's head popped out—everyone was excited, and *I* got so excited I asked if it was a boy or a girl before the body was even out!

It only took a few more minutes and a few more pushes, and out she came, screaming like a wild banshee. We had a quiet, mellow name picked out for a girl, but that changed as soon as we saw and heard her.

The placenta slipped right out, which was a good feeling. In fact, the whole birthing experience was a good feeling. I had actually delivered our baby without any drugs, just kind, reassuring help from my husband, midwife and doctor.

Bill laid the baby on my stomach, and we called in Trina, my twelve-year-old stepdaughter, to see her new little sister, Callie Marie. Trina was so happy she started to cry. Bill let Spike cut the umbilical cord and hold Callie while he stitched me. I had torn a little right where my old episiotomy scar was, and I needed two stitches.

My sister, speaking from experience, had warned me that second babies come faster than first ones, but I had never dreamed it would happen that fast. I was admitted into the hospital at 1:15 p.m., and Callie was born at 1:38. The nurse told me I had broken the hospital record. My total length of labor was eight and a half hours, with one and a half hours of active labor.

While I was holding our new baby girl, admiring her and watching her nurse, Spike figured it was a good time to tell me how he had gotten back so fast. It had never dawned on me that he would have missed the whole birth if he had driven back. He told me that there were so many stops for road work that he had gotten very nervous thinking he wouldn't make it in time. So he drove to the closest airport and chartered a plane home. I thought he was joking, but he was serious. He decided to tell me after it was all over so I wouldn't worry about the money he had spent for the plane. Thank you, dear.

I teased him about being so dramatic, but I really was glad he made it there in time to share and enjoy this wonderful experience, just as we had planned for so many months.

*Judy now lives in Sacramento with her children and works as an account executive for a country-western radio station. She writes, "Callie is a very unique child and heads always turn when she's around. I am enjoying watching her grow up, and I feel good about her start in life."*

# The Clinic Baby

by Mary Cooper

---

One month before my due date I went to see the obstetrician who had delivered my son Martin two years previously. Although I was planning a homebirth, I wanted to reestablish rapport with him in case I might need to go to the hospital. After examining me, he said I was 2 to 3 centimeters dilated, and he expected me to give birth within a week.

The next day I lost some of the mucus plug, which sent me into a tailspin. I didn't have anything ready for the homebirth, so I bought all the supplies I needed, sterilized a birth pack, and got the baby's bed ready. All this preparation took several days.

The next week when I went in for my regular prenatal appointment at the Clinic, I was still 2 to 3 centimeters dilated and expecting to start labor at any moment. I was uncomfortable and couldn't sleep well. I was having Braxton-Hicks contractions often but not in a regular pattern. The following week at my checkup I was *still* 2 to 3 centimeters and nothing was happening!

When Kate checked me the next week, I was 4 centimeters dilated. She said, "Any time now!" I felt like I was walking around with a basketball between my legs. By this time I had resterilized the birth pack twice. The warmup contractions were getting more frequent but were still not regular. I felt past ready!

The next week, exactly one month after seeing the obstetrician, I went to the Clinic, and Kate and I had a long talk which eased my mind. She said she wouldn't do a pelvic exam since that was getting us too excited all along—the baby would come when it was ready. I agreed! As I was getting up, I had a contraction. Then as I was getting dressed, I had another one, stronger than any I had had so far. Kate said to come back in the afternoon if they kept up, and she'd check me.

As I was going down the hall, I had another contraction. I made an appointment for the next week, and I had another one. As I was paying my bill, I had another one. When I took Martin to the bathroom, I had another one. As I was about to walk out the door, I experienced a contraction so strong that I had to sit down. Mary, one of the midwives, saw me and suggested that I call Mike, my husband. While explaining the situation to Mike, I was doing slow deep breathing. He said he'd be right over to drive me home so we could prepare for the birth. After I hung up, Mary timed the contractions. They were five minutes apart and a minute long.

At 11:10 a.m. I went to an examining room, and Kate checked me after a contraction. She said I was 8 centimeters dilated. She wanted to check me during a contraction to see if there was any difference. Mike came in while Kate was examining me the second time. She said, "You're 8 . . . no, 9 . . . no, 10 centimeters dilated!" She said we could go to a friend's house nearby, or to the hospital, or, if we really wanted to, we could stay where we were. I said that if I couldn't go home, I wanted to stay at the Clinic.

My contractions were coming very rapidly and getting intense. My back was feeling a lot of pressure. Kate got a blanket to wrap around me so I could walk discreetly from the examining room to the yoga room, which was being set up with massage tables and lots of pillows for the birth. I felt past caring about modesty. Walking was difficult, but it felt good to be off my back. I had a contraction while I was standing, and it was easier. I decided to get on my hands and knees. The contractions were one on top of the other now and it seemed like there was no break at all between them. Kate and Lorraine didn't want me to push, so Mike and Mary kept telling me, "Blow! Blow! Blow!" But I pushed a little anyway since it was such an overpowering sensation. When I did, the bag of water broke all over Kate. I could feel her wet sleeve on my leg. She didn't mind, but I thought of her having to spend the rest of the day in wet clothes.

From that point on, it seemed like a long series of contractions with no letup. I wondered how long it could go on and if I would be able to stand it. I wanted to shriek, but Lorraine said, "Keep it low, low like a cow." So I said, "Oh, oh," as low in my throat as I could. It felt so good, I kept on even when a contraction ended. I began to feel suffocated, as if I couldn't get enough air. Then I felt a stinging sensation all through my bottom and heavy pressure by my clitoris. This truly hurt, but it was over so quickly, it was really nothing. After three more contractions, the head was crowning. Everyone was saying, "Blow! Don't push! Blow, blow!" Then everyone was excited and I kept asking, "What's happening down there?" They told me the head was out. Pretty soon out popped the body. What a relief!

The baby was not crying. I asked several times if she was all

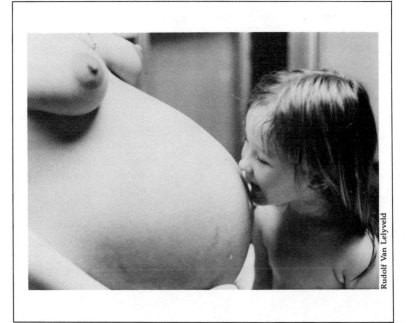

Rudolf Van Lelyveld

right. "Yes, she's fine," someone replied. I thought, She! It *is* a girl! Oh Misty! And then she started to cry—it was 12:04 p.m. Kate cut the cord so I could get off my hands and knees. I felt very out of it, and Misty was an awful blue color. Kate suctioned her and since the Clinic wasn't prepared for births, finding something to wrap her in wasn't easy. Finally, someone in the waiting room gave us a blanket.

Martin had quietly observed the birth. He was full of questions and wondered why Misty was all wet and why "they (the midwives) put water all over her." We all stayed and relaxed for a few hours, enjoying the special treatment. Misty's color improved by the time we were ready to go home.

So, that is the story of how Misty was born in seventy minutes at the Clinic. The next week we donated a gown and a shirt to be kept on hand for such emergencies.

*Four and a half years prior to her first pregnancy, Mary had emergency surgery to remove an ovarian cyst. One ovary and half of a tube were removed from one side and a wedge section was done on the remaining ovary. During the surgery, the intact tube was also damaged. After several years of infertility testing, she was told that she only had a 1 percent chance of having a viable pregnancy. She now has two healthy children and teaches gymnastics classes for young children. She lives with her family in a home she describes as "permanently under construction." On their twenty acres she raises produce, pigs and a pony. She hopes to open a school of gymnastics some day.*

# Ready or Not

## Pam Morhmann

---

Our baby was due in early May, rose-blooming time. We planned to welcome her quietly and gently at home, with our son Zach sharing in her birth. There would be bouquets from the garden and a close friend or two. After the birth, the babe would nurse, and we would lie together quietly. Common enough expectations.

It was with surprise, then, and a stab of panic that I realized my water had broken a full ten weeks before my due date. Ironically, my husband Dave and I were at the Clinic having just attended a childbirth education class that dealt with premature labor. Somewhere in my mind a voice repeated with growing intensity, It's too early! I remember remaining icily calm, probably because none of what was happening seemed the least bit real. I was soon surrounded by the midwives and my husband, his eyes so large and round in a face gone white—my own fear staring back at me.

What followed was three hours of bureaucratic indecision about where I should be taken—air transport to a large city hospital or ambulance to a local hospital that was equipped to handle such a premature birth. During that time I felt only painless uterine tightening. It was almost possible to convince myself it would all go away, and this baby would remain cradled within until May. I received loving encouragement and support from those around me, their mouths offering words of comfort and concern that my mind could only partially register. I was being drawn more and more inward towards my baby, trying to surround her with my love and protect her from what lay ahead. Nothing seemed to promise that it would be easy.

Five hours after my water had broken, I found myself in an ambulance on my way to a small hospital forty-five miles away. The very word "premature" rattled around in my head, and I prodded it, foreign as it was to me. I had not read the section on premature birth in my childbirth books, never dreaming it would happen to me. I had never known anyone who had given birth prematurely. Stranger in a strange land with nothing solid or real.

Once in the hospital, I was started on an IV, and Ritodrine was administered to try to stop my labor. My contractions remained mild, about four minutes apart. I was 2 centimeters dilated. When the doctor arrived, I wanted him to tell me what might happen and what my baby's chance to live was. I didn't want my mind creating a situation worse than what could actually occur. I wanted to be prepared. I was told that a baby born at thirty-one weeks gestation had an 80 percent chance of survival. The major concern would be the condition of the lungs. If they were insufficiently developed there could be respiratory distress syndrome or Hyaline Membrane Disease, either of which could decrease her chance of survival. I was also told that because she was in the breech position, I would be given a cesarean section so as not to put undue stress on her fragile spinal cord.

Dave and I held hands—it was actually more like clinging. We told each other that this baby was strong and healthy and that all would be well. We buoyed each other up as we watched the clock and the fetal monitor. We made light conversation with the nurse, wondering all the while if my labor would stop, if our baby would be healthy, if I would really need a cesarean section. I remember hearing the babies crying in the nursery across the hall and wanting to close the sound out. Those cries made me aware of my fear that my baby wouldn't survive.

An hour and a half later it was obvious that the Ritodrine was not going to work. My labor was progressing, and our baby would be born soon. The doctor came in at one point to check me, and his face registered a subtle change. "The baby has turned," he said. He checked and rechecked, finally admitting, "If I hadn't felt it with my own hands, I wouldn't have believed it." Our relief was sudden and soothing—no cesarean! Our baby seemed to be working with us, and our feelings of encouragement were great. All would certainly be well.

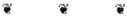

4:00 a.m.: I'm checked and told I'm 4 centimeters dilated. Suddenly the contractions double, triple in strength. They have a power to tear me apart. I am overwhelmed by the sudden intensity. Viselike I grip Dave's neck and shoulders, grabbing for support. And then I feel the baby's head coming. Coming! A mad race down the hall to the delivery room. Dave's voice shouting, "Blow! Blow!" My cheeks puffing in and out with such force that even hours later they prickle from the exertion. A quick lift onto the delivery table with no time to get my legs into the awkward stirrups. Our baby's head is born and seconds later her body emerges.

❧        ❧        ❧

At 4:14 a.m., March 4, Rosanne Elizabeth made her hurried entrance, weighing a slight three pounds. Most birth stories end at about this point, but ours was only beginning. Rosanne was to remain in the hospital for the next six weeks. Her birth was the beginning of a strange and often difficult time until we were able to bring her home.

We were lucky that she had no lung problems. Three hours after birth she was off oxygen, which was extremely encouraging. Her lungs seemed strong and healthy for her tiny size. Seeing her for the first time was a shock. She lay in her isolette looking so fragile and vulnerable. It's hard to explain the feelings that raced through me, except to say that I loved her intensely and immediately wanted to spare her any pain. I wanted to take her in my arms and rock her, welcome her, somehow reassure her. Instead, I put my hand through the porthole of the isolette and hesitantly stroked her hand. I felt oddly intimidated by her, by her very smallness. On her body were attached cardiac monitor lead wires, a temperature probe and an umbilical catheter. Her face was bruised a deep purple. Her arms and legs were encased in skin too big to fit. I sat and stroked her and tried to convince myself she was mine.

It took a few days for me to adjust to my daughter. Watching her lying in the isolette with wires attached here and there, seeing the nurses handle her with such calm assurance, I felt alienated and isolated from her. I felt jealous of the mothers who could hold their babies, nurse them, and then wheel gloriously out the doors with them to take up normal lives. Those days in the beginning were hard—a time of adjustment and shifting of gears.

Slowly I became part of my daughter's life. From the day she was born I began using an electric breast pump to express milk every three hours, day and night. Beginning with just a few drops of colostrum, all was meticulously saved so that Rosanne, although unable to nurse, received my milk right from the start. At first she was fed through a tube, and weeks later she was able to start drinking from a bottle. The nurses, whom I made it a point to get to know, understood my feelings and were an important factor in making me comfortable around my baby. I asked innumerable questions, and they took the time to explain how the monitors worked, what the particular notations in Rosanne's chart stood for, and the basic elements of her care. Their empathy and loving support were instrumental in helping Dave and me come to feel so

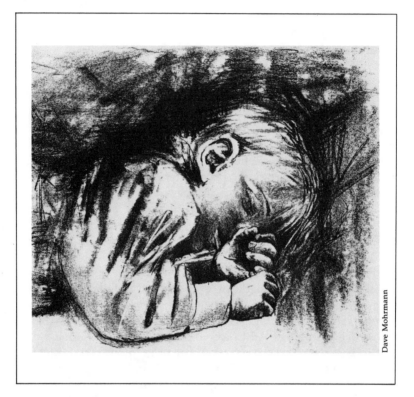

Dave Mohrmann

at home in the nursery.

While I was still in the hospital, Dave and I would go to the nursery every hour or so and sit by the isolette, hands through the portholes, stroking her back, her leg, her hand. We learned to stimulate her by tapping the soles of her feet or rocking her water-filled mattress whenever she had an apnea or bradycardia spell (common occurences in preemies, in which the infant forgets to breathe or the heart rate slows). Sometimes her heart rate would slow to the point that it would set off an alarm, and she would need more vigorous prodding or perhaps a whiff of oxygen. At those times my heart would pound and my stomach clench, and her fragility would confront me again.

At two weeks of age, Rosanne began having increasingly frequent apnea spells. The alarm on her cardiac monitor filled the air like a scream. All day we sat by her, watching the monitor and stroking her. My fear was like a lump in my stomach. Tests were

ordered and an x-ray machine appeared, looking large and ominous. People moved about with quiet efficiency. I cried in a nurse's
arms with tension and a building fear and frustration. There is a
deep sense of helplessness watching your sick baby cared for by
others, not being able to cuddle her and rock her and let her know
you're there. Test results trickled in, all of them negative. There
was no infection; her lungs were clear. Rosanne's apnea seemed to
be stemming purely from the immaturity of her nervous system.
We watched and waited.

By the second day it was obvious she was beginning to need
help breathing. First she was given oxygen, but when that didn't
provide enough help, she was put on a respirator. My heart ached
as I watched her. What must this world that she had hurried into
seem like to her? I had a strong impulse to grab her and run
somewhere dark and quiet, and rock, soothe and hold her tight.
We were restless and slept little that night. I dreamed of large black
tubes with strong suction attacking me as I clung to a piling in the
middle of the ocean, my vulnerability and fear coming through to
me even in sleep.

When we arrived at the hospital the next morning, we found
Rosanne off the respirator and breathing on her own. The crisis
had passed as quickly as it had begun.

Our days fell into a pattern that wasn't always easy to live with.
I drove the forty-five miles to the hospital at least five mornings a
week, returning in the late afternoon in time to pump my milk,
cook dinner, and collapse into bed. Dave tried to make the trip
with me at least two days a week, whatever his work schedule
would allow. I felt torn between Rosanne and our home life. Since
the bulk of my energy was going to Rosanne, Dave and Zach were
feeling somewhat left out. Dave felt frustrated at not being able to
spend more time with his new daughter. It was hard hearing only
verbal reports from me after having been so involved with her birth
and first few days. As for Zach, his new sister was a small person
connected to wires, living in a plastic box, whom he had to look
at through a pane of glass. It was not an easy time for any of us.
The very hardest moments for me were awaking in the night and
wanting to hold my baby. When I pumped my milk in the middle
of the night, I would close my eyes and imagine it was really
Rosanne nursing at my breast.

With premature babies you learn to cheer about any small progress—a weight gain of even half an ounce or an increase in the

amount of milk taken and retained. There was the day we were finally able to hold her. The day she was able to start "nippling" (drinking from a bottle). The day she graduated from the isolette to an open crib. The day I arrived to find the cardiac monitor no longer attached to her body. The nurses cheered right along with us. They became special friends, actually our extended family. We felt their love and caring wash over all of us. On Rosanne's one-month birthday, as we strolled her around the nursery, our paper gowns crackling, we were surprised by a chorus of "Happy Birthday" and a cake with one candle that the head nurse had made. It was another example of their thoughtfulness and sharing of our joy.

Finally, the day came when we were able to take her home, one day short of her six-week birthday. She weighed four pounds, nine and a half ounces. Her cheeks had become chubby, her knees round. I felt elated and at the same time a little scared. She had been cared for in a very controlled environment for almost six weeks. I found myself wondering: Would I keep her warm enough? Would she thrive? That first night I lay awake listening to all of her squeaks, grunts and sighs, getting to know my baby in our home environment. From then on, my fear fell away, and I totally relaxed for the first time since she was born. We delighted in being a family together at last. Zach's sister became real for him, and he beamed as he held her or rubbed her back.

She is now almost eight weeks old. She still isn't nursing, finding breastfeeding difficult and frustrating after the "preemie" nipples. But we try once or twice a day and as she continues to grow and gain strength, nursing will be another thing she will accomplish if we're patient enough.

Although our original expectations regarding Rosanne's birth weren't met, in a way they were surpassed—through the caring, concern and gentleness we encountered from everyone connected with Rosanne's care, and the feeling, close to triumph, that we felt when we finally brought her home as part of our family.

*After overcoming their initial difficulties, Rosanne and Pam had a successful two-year nursing career. Pam now teaches at a local elementary school. Dave is an artist and writer. Pam's interests include gardening and photography.*

# Satish's and Tomas' Births

Lindy Thorpe

My first child was born in a hospital. It was such a horrifying experience that when I conceived again, nine years later, I was scared. I didn't know what to expect.

A friend of mine, Alison, who was just beginning her training as a midwife, told me about the midwives at the Clinic. I went and met them—their smiles and warmth were most welcome. My husband George, my daughter Allison and I attended the birthing classes. The prenatal yoga classes were a big help throughout my pregnancy. We decided to have a homebirth. Since we live back in the hills, we thought it would be safer than trying to drive down to the hospital.

We were all ready for the big day. It was the end of October, and I was 2 centimeters dilated. Lorraine told me it could be any time. Then, a month later, on November 28, Lorraine told me I was 4 centimeters dilated. Again, it could be any time. I was really depressed, and the anxiety was driving me nuts.

Finally, on November 30, I woke up with little cramps. George was ready to go to work. I told him, "I think this could be it, but I'm not sure." I'd had so many false starts that I'd given up and accepted the fact that I was going to be pregnant forever. He left to get the midwives and our breathing coach. They all arrived around 7:30 a.m.

My labor was so different than I had imagined. The contractions were mild. Everything glowed and the colors around me were bright. I never thought having a baby could be such a high. We sat on the bed, talking and laughing between contractions. It was like a slumber party. My daughter stayed home from school that day. Her charge was to take pictures and write down the time of birth. It was great to be able to share the birth with her, especially since she wanted to be part of it.

At 11:30 a.m., Lorraine checked me. I was 8 centimeters dilated. I couldn't believe I had dilated so much with such mild contractions. She advised George and me to go for a walk to help me progress further. Sure enough, it worked. We walked about fifty

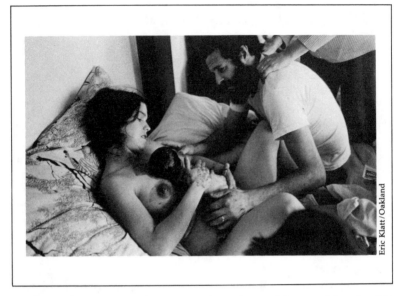

Eric Klatt/Oakland

yards, and my contractions started coming quicker and harder. We headed back to the house.

While we were gone, Alison and Lorraine had set up the bed and their instruments. I knew it wouldn't be long until I would finally hold my son. (I knew it was a boy from a dream I had had when I first conceived. A man in my dream told me I'd have a boy and that I would name him Satish. Later, a sonogram confirmed that it was indeed a boy. We saw his little testicles on the screen. What an experience that was!)

Lorraine had a hard time breaking the bag of water. It seemed like I pushed forever, but after his head came through, which really burned, his little body slipped right out. What a great sensation! He made his appearance at 1:16 p.m. He was so beautiful. His coloring was pink, and he looked like a little angel.

My daughter had been too involved with me to take pictures, but Alison took a few. Lorraine was beautiful, so calm and relaxed throughout the whole birth. She really helped me to stay in tune with myself and my body.

The high that came afterwards was wonderful. I glowed, beamed and wanted the whole world to come and see my new baby boy, Satish.

❦          ❦          ❦

My second son was born at home twenty-one months later. His birthing was special, too. I went to the Clinic for my prenatal care and attended yoga classes twice a week. I was in good shape and not scared or nervous as I had been with Satish. This time I wanted a girl and thought for sure it was because I carried "her" so differently than I had Satish. I even bought pink diaper pins.

We really wanted Lorraine and Alison to help bring this baby into our world, but Lorraine was leaving for two weeks at the beginning of August, which was the same time as my due date. In desperation I took castor oil for three days at the end of July. I'd start to get contractions, but nothing ever happened.

Lorraine was gone. We talked to Alison, and she recommended Kate. I had seen her working with Alison at a friend's birth, and liked her. So George and I agreed on Kate.

On Sunday morning, August 9, around 8 o'clock, I started having mild contractions. I told a friend who was visiting, and she started timing them. They were so irregular I didn't tell George about them until 11:00 a.m. He was all ready to go play baseball. At first he thought I was kidding, trying to get him to stay home. When he realized I wasn't, he left to get the midwives.

My sister and another friend arrived. It was hot, so we spent most of the day sitting in the front yard in the shade, doing laundry and talking. It was fun trying to guess when the next contraction was going to come.

Kate and Alison, with her daughter Kali, arrived around 3:00 p.m. They checked me, and I was 6 centimeters dilated. The time seemed to be going fast.

Another friend arrived with her baby. My Allison was there, too. She was to take pictures ("This time, I promise," she told me, and she did take some nice ones). Satish was in a very good mood all day. He seemed to sense what was going on. I was feeling high and excited about meeting my new "daughter."

Kate told George and me to go for a walk. We did and it was hot. But it was nice to get away from everyone to spend some time alone. While we were walking, my water broke. All of a sudden, a gush of water splattered all over—it scared me. Everyone in the house heard it, and Kate and Alison came outside to see what had happened. We went back in the house and set everything up. The bed was made up in the living room where it was cooler and everyone could participate.

The contractions were getting stronger and closer together.

Whenever I thought I was going to lose control of my breathing, I'd look up at my guru's picture—just looking into his eyes made it easier for me.

The time came to push. After a few good pushes, the head came out. But the shoulders were stuck. Kate knew just what to do. She told me to get on my knees. "You're kidding," I said. George didn't hesitate. He picked me up and put me on my knees. (What strength!)

I pushed with everything I had, then Kate told Alison, "Get the scissors." I pushed again, but this time I felt I had help from my guru. All of a sudden, out the baby came—no scissors. Kate had Alison get the oxygen ready in case we needed it.

It was 6:45 p.m. when he arrived, all blue. I heard Allison say, "It's a boy!" I felt disappointed, but when I realized he was having trouble breathing, he was so blue and limp, I cried and prayed for my baby. At that point I didn't care whether it was a boy or a girl.

Kate was wonderful. She was so calm and fast. She did everything: mouth to mouth, rubbed him and talked to him. It was beautiful to watch her. She got him breathing, then put the oxygen on him. They worked on him for a couple of hours, getting his color back and removing the mucus from his lungs. Everyone was praying and telling him, "Come on and breathe." It was great to feel so much energy going towards my new son. I was ecstatic when I could finally hold him and I thanked God, our divine Mother, for giving him to us.

He was nine pounds, nine ounces, twenty-one inches long—a truly big boy with a head of black hair. We named him Tomas Walsh. I felt high after this birth too, and wanted everyone to come and see this beautiful new human being who decided to stay with us after all.

It was really great to experience two births at home. Now I understand why my mother had so many children—eleven, including four sets of twins. All the midwives helped to make my childbirth memories very special. I'll never forget them and what they did for us.

*Lindy is now raising her three children as a single parent and working at a local inn. She continues to follow the teachings of Paramahansa Yogananda and loves to write, dance and practice yoga in her spare time.*

# An Adoptive Birth

by Ruthanne Bassett

An adoptive birth is quite different from a natural birth, but the result is the same, a beautiful child who makes a family grow.

In March my husband Quentin and I decided to find a baby to adopt. We had put a lot of thought into adoption and realized that we wanted an infant. The agencies told us that it would be a long wait, without much hope of a newborn. Despite this discouraging outlook, we were determined to find our child. Looking to God for encouragement, we made prayer and belief our tools to success. We began talking and writing to everyone we knew about our desire to find a child.

In August my mother located our baby. She'd put out feelers and had learned a lot about independent adoptions where the birth parents and the adoptive parents get together without the help of an agency. One Sunday afternoon, as she was doing volunteer work in a medical information booth at a county fair, she was approached by a young woman who said she was four and a half months pregnant and wanted to put the baby up for adoption.

Mom phoned us immediately and informed me, "I've found your baby."

The words took a long time to sink in. A week or two later I began to realize that we were going to get a child in four months. I knew that the waiting would be difficult and not without challenges. I called these months of waiting, "correspondence pregnancy." Alice, the natural mother, was almost a thousand miles away in San Diego. In addition to our concern for her health and happiness, curiosity led us to meet her in September. After that we wrote and phoned back and forth. Alice had a lot of problems which we shared across the miles. There were many emotional ups and downs.

I decided to try to breastfeed our baby. That decision demanded continual physical, mental and spiritual efforts on my part. I adapted my diet and began preparing myself. After a month of stimulating my breasts I was able to express droplets of milk.

We began building, borrowing and buying in anticipation of a larger family. My friends gave me a baby shower. Alison, one of the midwives from the Clinic, spent time with us, answering our questions and sharing her knowledge of newborn care. We read, discussed ideas, talked with other parents and waited.

December was long and rainy. The due date was vague so we were alert for a phone call by the second week. On Christmas Eve, we drove to San Francisco and spent Christmas with our families. Alice kept in touch with us daily via the phone. It was so hard to wait that we finally decided to fly to San Diego. Just as we were leaving for the airport, Alice called to say that she was going to the hospital.

As we began our journey, I could only think about the baby who was going to come into our family. I watched the children at the airport (Christmas is such a family time). We boarded the plane, ate nuts and drank soda, then debarked. We took a cab to the hotel where we received a message that Alice had gone home from the hospital—a false alarm.

At 4:30 the next morning, Alice's roommate called to say that she was on her way to the hospital again. Sleepily we got dressed and called for a taxi. It was dark as we approached the hospital with its giant stork guarding the women's pavilion. A nurse in the lobby directed me to the labor room but wouldn't let Quentin in.

I spent the next three hours coaching Alice before I held our baby in my arms. I wished I had read more about labor and delivery. There was a machine that monitored the baby's heartbeat and the mother's contractions. A nurse bustled in and out regularly. I prayed for, talked to and coached Alice. She was uncomfortable and had an epidural anesthesia two hours before the delivery. The doctor came in now and then to check her and talk with the nurse. Finally they handed me a blue paper suit, including hat and shoes, and told me to wait while they prepped her for the birth. Then the nurse led me into the delivery room and offered me a stool about ten feet behind the doctor.

"Now stay back there and don't get in his way," she warned.

I sat, practically in a daze. I prayed for the baby and an easy delivery. Everything around me was so unfamiliar. The doctor put together what I guessed were forceps. He inserted the forceps and pulled. It didn't really seem possible that the bloody ball I saw was a baby's head.

"Can you push now?" asked the doctor.

She must have, because out came a little face. I saw movement and heard a cry.

"You've got a baby girl," said the doctor.

We had all been thinking it would be a boy.

"Is that OK, Ru?" asked Alice.

I couldn't believe my eyes. It was here, a baby girl. The doctor cut the cord very efficiently and gave the child to the nurse. It was hard to contain myself but I stayed on my stool as she wiped the baby with a towel and put her under a heat lamp on the other side of the room. I didn't see the rest of the birth because my eyes were on the baby. After a few minutes the nurse said, "You can hold her now."

I thought about breastfeeding as I walked across the room. The nurse put her into my arms. She was so tiny. Her skin was white and peeling; she had no hair but was very beautiful. I held her for a minute, then asked if it was all right to put her to my breast. The doctor stopped stitching for a minute and looked up questioningly.

I explained, "I'm going to try to breastfeed her. I can already express some milk."

"Go ahead if you want," he replied, shrugging with doubt.

I pulled up the paper shirt and turned the little mouth toward my breast. Her lips touched the nipple, she latched on and started to suck.

Alice asked to see the baby. I showed it to her somewhat hesitantly. I didn't want her to change her mind.

"You guys will give her a good home," she said wearily.

Later the nurse let Quentin and me share a few private moments in the labor room with our little baby before leading us to the nursery. She handed the newborn to another nurse who efficiently began to handle her. As I reached the doorway she commanded, "You've got to scrub before you come in here."

"What are you going to do with her?" I asked.

"Just check her over, give her some water to make sure she can suck."

"Are you going to put silver nitrate in her eyes?"

"Of course." She turned to our baby, busily measuring her head. "Come back this afternoon, then you can have her."

I was disappointed, but I could tell there was nothing we could do to change hospital routine. Although I really didn't want to let the baby out of my sight, I was tired.

"Come on," said Quentin. "We'll come back later. Let's eat breakfast. Maybe we can go back to the hotel and sleep."

When we returned that afternoon, we scrubbed and put on smocks. They offered me a chair at the back of the nursery, then a nurse handed our baby to me. She was so tiny and delicate that it was awkward to hold her and put her to my breast. She sucked hard for a few minutes. Then I tried the other breast. She sucked a while, then seemed to be sleeping.

"Don't you want to give her a bottle?" asked the nurse.

"No, I'm going to breastfeed her," I said.

"But did she get anything?"

"Well, uh . . . " I stammered. "I didn't think that mattered so much the first couple of days."

"Well, what are you going to do then?" she asked.

"I have this Lact-aid nurser kit." I showed her the box with rings, tubes and disposable pouches.

"I've never heard of that before. You'd better talk to my supervisor."

The supervisor walked over quickly. "I'll call your pediatrician and see what he wants to do," she said.

The doctor was very encouraging on the phone. He said he knew a nurse-practitioner who had experience with the Lact-aid and that he would make arrangements for her to come to the hospital that evening and help us.

I nursed our baby again that afternoon, then the nurse-practitioner showed us how to fill the Lact-aids and hold the tiny tube to my breast. It was awkward to get coordinated with the baby, but she drank some formula and we noticed some droplets of my milk.

After the 10:00 p.m. feeding we went back to the hotel for the night, exhausted. The next morning we returned, and we were told that we could take Rachel home that afternoon as long as we promised to see a doctor the following day, New Year's Eve.

We left the hospital when she was two days old and began our trek home. Our first stop would be the Clinic. Inclement weather delayed our flight for two hours. We waited quietly at the crowded boarding gate with our tiny bundle before boarding the flight to San Francisco. During takeoff and landing, I offered her my breast, but she sleepily rejected it.

It was still raining in San Francisco where Quentin's brother met us and drove us to their parents' home. Rachel slept in a large suitcase that first long night away from the hospital. She woke up three or four times, and I groggily struggled to coordinate the Lact-aid, my breast and her mouth. I was exhausted the next morning.

We left early in order to make our 2:00 p.m. appointment at the Clinic. It was raining hard as we strapped our little one into her car seat and began the long drive. Roadwork held us up, but we made it to our appointment with ten minutes to spare. The nor-

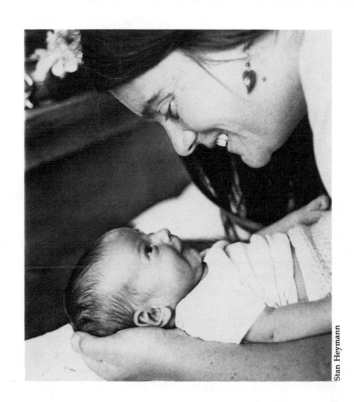

Stan Heymann

mally bustling Clinic was deserted.

She was weighed, measured, listened to, poked and prodded. We talked with Kate about the birth and asked questions about the next few days of caring for our baby. After receiving a good report, we made one last stop at the store for formula and supplies. Then we drove the ten miles to our cold, empty home.

Before long, Quentin had a fire blazing. I fed Rachel. It was getting easier. From San Diego to our home in Northern California, a thousand miles in three days: planes, cars and pouring rain. Rachel is at home now with us, and we are a family.

*Ruthanne and her husband have adopted a second baby. They say, "Our success in adoption is due to an active prayer life and confidence in God." They are associated with a biblical research and teaching fellowship and feel that their entire family thrives on their Christian lifestyle.*

# Expectations, Disappointments and Perfect Moments

by Peg Anderson

I became pregnant the first time we tried, and I seemed to start expanding immediately. By the time I was six months pregnant, people were saying, "Any day now, eh?" I had been having dreams of more than one baby, occasionally interspersed with very vivid dreams of a lively baby girl.

My husband Harris and I were planning a homebirth. My midwives were concerned about the possibility of twins, so they asked that I get a sonogram. I, too, was very curious. One hour before the appointment for the sonogram I drank the required amount of water to expand my bladder, enabling the radiologist to get a better picture of the fetus. The doctor started scanning my belly and almost immediately diagnosed a complete placenta previa. The placenta was covering my cervix, making it impossible for me to deliver my baby vaginally. Also, there was just one baby.

Dazed, I went to the bathroom, not willing to accept this. When I returned I only had to look at my midwife and Harris to know it was true. I burst into tears, realizing that all our plans were instantly changed and that I would be bringing my baby into a very different environment from the one I had imagined.

Harris and I had to go through a grieving process for a week or so. We had actually been anticipating twins in addition to the romanticism of a home delivery. Interestingly, two weeks before the sonogram I had dreamt that I delivered a beautiful baby girl. I had no experience of labor, and when I looked down, I saw two incisions across my abdomen.

Our immediate task was to find an obstetrician to do the cesarean. We located a good one, and he soon made us aware of the seriousness of my condition. Most women with placenta previa experience heavy bleeding around the sixth month and have to be confined to bed. The bleeding is caused by the placenta separating from the wall of the expanding uterus. This, of course, seriously threatens the fetus' source of oxygen and can kill the mother if the bleeding is profuse. By this time I was seven and a half months pregnant and had experienced no bleeding. We live sixty miles from the hospital and our doctor said that if the placenta started separating we might not have time to ensure the safety of both the baby and me. He suggested we move into a motel within five minutes of the hospital. We made the move in my thirty-fifth week and were lucky to find acquaintances who gave us the use of a spare bedroom in their home.

After a week of very tense waiting, the doctor said, "Why wait for an emergency?" He wanted me to have an amniocentesis to determine the maturity of the baby's lungs, and if they were mature, he would "take" the baby. The amniocentesis made me very nervous. I could feel the blood drain from my face as the needle went in. I felt as if my baby and I were being invaded. The doctor noticed blood in the fluid sample, which meant the placenta had begun to detach. We waited nervously for the results the next morning, September 7. Finally, toward noon, the results of the test were ready—the lungs were mature enough for the baby to be born. My due date was September 23, so the delivery would be more than two weeks early.

I went right to the hospital, was hooked up to the fetal heart monitor and was prepared for surgery. Harris was with me throughout this time, literally my body guard. Several weeks previously he had taken a class on procedure for cesarean births, so he knew what to expect.

The birth was scheduled for 4:30 p.m. I was wheeled down the hall—scared, excited, but in control. What followed was the most difficult part of the whole birth. I was settled on the operating table and right away fitted with a catheter—spreadeagled on the table, head tilted down. I started to shake. The catheter burned horribly, the doctor was late, and I ended up spending forty minutes in this position. The anesthesiologist gave me some Valium though I protested weakly. Harris was not allowed to be with me before the actual surgery, so I was very alone with my fears.

Finally the doctor arrived, but before he could begin the surgery he had to doublecheck my placenta's position by inserting his finger through the cervix. If I started to bleed, I would immediately be put under general anesthesia, something I did not want to happen. He checked my placenta, and though it was painful, I did not bleed. I felt my use of visualization in the past weeks had let my body know what I wanted and didn't want it to do.

I was rolled over on my side for an epidural injection which would deaden feeling from the chest down but allow me to see my baby right away. To my great relief Harris was then allowed to come and sit by me. A pleasant calm came over me almost immediately from the injection, and my shaking stopped. I kept my eyes on Harris' face as he watched the procedure.

The doctors began working very fast; I was only aware of a prodding motion. Afterward, Harris described how they pulled layers of me apart and reached in to locate the baby. The doctor caught a foot through the membrane, but it pulled away from him. The membrane was pierced and bloody fluid sprayed out. The doctor then pulled out what Harris described later as an ominous battleship-gray-colored little body. Thank God he didn't betray his fears at that moment. The baby was rushed to the warming table, and I heard a strong little yelp. Harris watched as circles of pink grew on our little girl's cheeks.

I kept repeating Harris' name out of my need for information. I was very calm, instinctively knowing everything was all right, but so impatient to see her. Then she was brought over to me wrapped up tightly in a blanket, so absolutely beautiful. I said, "Harris, she has your mouth!" He then took her to the nursery while I went into recovery. The nurse there had to push and prod my uterus, an extremely painful procedure, but that was secondary to my joy. Finally, after an hour, I was reunited with my daughter who began eagerly nursing. It was a perfect moment; I was in love.

*Peg, who has lived in Northern California for eleven years, previously resided in Minnesota, Mexico and parts of Europe. Her teenaged son Rio, her baby daughter Sophia and the home she and her husband have been building for the past five years keep her busy. She also owns a natural food and health care store which she finds satisfying, challenging and occasionally very trying. Peg says, "I am currently practicing doing absolutely nothing at certain times and find it deeply fulfilling."*

# Our Three Sons

by Kathy Sargent

The births of our three sons were as different as day and night. With our first, I was young and naive. I didn't think anything could ever go wrong, so I was very relaxed about the pregnancy and birth.

Everett and I had planned our first child—we would have him one year and nine months after we were married. We attended Lamaze classes and learned about the birth process, breathing, exercises, relaxation techniques and what each of our jobs would be. What a different approach to childbirth from our parents! Strange how we have to be trained to do something so natural.

At 4:00 one morning, two weeks past my due date, I was awakened by something warm and wet—my water had broken. All at once it was everywhere. Everett called the hospital, and we were told to come in when my contractions were harder and closer together.

At 1:00 p.m. we went to the hospital. I had moderate contractions until the late afternoon, then they got heavier. After every contraction I wanted ice—just the feel of it helped. Everett sat beside me, giving me ice and keeping me focused on the breathing. Whenever I started to tire out and say I couldn't go on, he was right there breathing with me. He really got me through it. I was given two shots of Demerol during the last stages, which slowed things down, and I rested awhile.

A few minutes before midnight, after I had been in the delivery room for an hour, the doctor decided to use forceps to get the baby out. I think he was superstitious because it was minutes from being Friday the thirteenth. I didn't really mind the forceps; I had been pushing a long time and was exhausted. I had used nearly every bit of strength I had. I was given an episiotomy, and Scott Everett was born at 11:55 p.m. after a twenty-hour labor. He weighed almost eight pounds. There was no damage from the forceps, just small red marks on each side of Scott's head which went away in a day or two.

I told friends afterwards, "It was the most thrilling thing I've

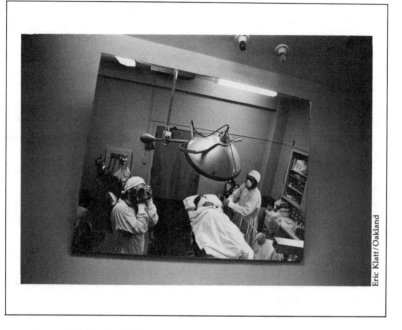

Eric Klatt/Oakland

ever done." I don't think it can ever be accurately described; it just has to be experienced.

   ❧     ❧     ❧

My second birth was my easiest. Labor started at 10:00 a.m. I went through all the stages pretty much "by the book." At one point during my labor when the contractions were getting hard, and I was beginning to wonder how long I could last, the doctor said I had quite a while to go, and went home to change a tire on his car. I think when you are told it will be a long time, you don't feel that you can keep going. If I had known it would only be a couple more hours, it would have seemed easier.

I was given one shot of Demerol and a small episiotomy. Wayne Bradley was born at 8:43 p.m., right on his due date. He weighed eight pounds, two ounces. I felt great after his delivery—my husband and I watched a movie and had dinner to celebrate.

   ❧     ❧     ❧

Our third son was my hardest. I went into labor cold and nervous, completely different from my two previous births. I couldn't stop shivering. It *was* the coldest night of the year, 26°, but even in warm rooms I was shaky. I began labor at 11:00 p.m.

with what felt like Braxton-Hicks contractions—they just continued longer, then quickly intensified. I think it was a harder labor because everything happened so quickly. I didn't have time to adjust to the different stages—each was there before I knew it. I had back labor, which I hadn't experienced before, and I didn't know how to deal with it. I felt like I was having contractions in front and in back, and I couldn't concentrate on both, so I kept losing the rhythm of my breathing. My husband was right there holding my hand, breathing with me and being very supportive. I can't imagine having only the cold metal handles of the delivery table to hold onto.

No drugs or episiotomy this time. The baby came so quickly I didn't have time to get properly situated on the delivery table. The stirrups were up so high, I was hardly touching the table, and no one would listen to me. I felt as if I was being ripped in two. Not at all like my other births.

Kevin James was born at 3:40 a.m., weighing six pounds, eight ounces. The doctor laid him on my tummy, and I remember touching his bluish leg and rubbing the soft ripples of his skin.

🐾     🐾     🐾

Would I give birth differently next time? I would like to try. I had always been frightened by homebirths. All the "what ifs?" ran through my mind. When I was asked to attend a friend's homebirth,* I felt apprehensive until I was reassured that my presence wouldn't have anything to do with whether or not anything went wrong.

It was a thrilling experience, and I can really appreciate why people choose to stay home. I think I would like to give birth in my own bed, wear (or not wear) what I want, and be able to shower afterwards and then have my baby right there with my whole family.

*After writing this story, Kathy sent the following note: "I am expecting again and after careful consideration, my husband and I decided we'll go to the hospital to have this one too. I was elated after attending the homebirth of my friend, but after the excitement wore off, and I found myself pregnant with the choice in front of me, I realized it wouldn't be for me." Kathy now has four sons and says she enjoys cutting hair and writing poetry.*

---

*See "Aurianna Miranda and Micah David," p. 156.

# One Ripe Cherry

by Jolynn Kottke

Because of bad luck and my inability to conform in a relationship, I found myself pregnant, single, and quite in lack of a nesting place. On the road I went, my wayward steps eventually leading me, through direct answer to my prayers, to the rural hills of Northern California. I found a mate in a sister, Abbie, and we shared twenty-four hours out of every day that followed; not lovers, but loving and learning and struggling on in our youthful fashion. Poor, but wealthy in soul.

The winter was unusually wet and two weeks prior to my due date the bridge on our road fell into the creek, leaving us cut off from the midwives—our strength, our hold on sanity. On Christmas Eve day, reminiscent of Mary and Joseph, we carried the birthing kit, blankets and bare necessities by horseback four miles to a cabin a friend generously offered. My due date came and went; that was when the real waiting began!

I thought I had gone through all the anxieties I needed to: my fears of a new lifestyle, coping with a child as a single mom, and general acceptance of the choices I had made. Abbie listened to it all, reassured and encouraged me. We went to birth classes together. We prayed, sang and danced the joy of this new life. Wood for the birth was stacked and ready, the birthing kit was sterilized, and we could hardly wait.

I continued to see a midwife weekly, but there was no evidence of the baby dropping into the birth position. Two weeks lagged by, then seventeen days. The midwives gave me so much support; tears flowed as we hashed and rehashed the situation and recounted my dates. Still, brows were furrowed. The midwives were justifiably concerned. When a baby is overdue, the placenta begins to break down, limiting the supply of nutrients and oxygen, especially during the stress of labor. The risks of stillborn or brain-damaged infants and maternal hemorrhaging are increased.

Doctor Bill gave us two arbitrary dates—if labor did not commence by January 20, he wanted the birth to take place at our local hospital rather than at home. If we failed to deliver by the twenty-fifth, he wanted me to go to a larger hospital equipped with a fetal heart monitor.

We tried everything. First the midwives gave me a tincture which I drank for a day and a half, to no avail. Next was a bottle of castor oil with orange juice; vigorous bowel movements are thought to stimulate the cervix, in hopes of inducing labor. It was a good purge but did not result in a single contraction. I wrote, I walked, I sang, I prayed, I let it all go. We started riding horses again, I chopped wood, I even rode the donkey the four miles home, falling off twice! Nothing stirred the yet-developing life inside me.

With a blur of emotion and anticipation, I had passed both dates set by Dr. Bill. We burned the birthing wood and just let go, realizing that the baby would decide when the birth would commence. My love for this child, whom I knew I was supposed to carry and bear, grew and the feeling that everything was all right grew along with it. I felt great! I could not believe I could feel so right and not be carrying something equally right.

On January 26, Mary took us to the hospital for a non-stress test. As a midwife and loving sister, her support aided us immeasurably. She explained that if the baby did not score well, it was unlikely that it would be able to handle the stress of labor. A cesarean section or an induced labor were becoming dreaded possibilities. It was pouring rain. I pressed my face against the cool glass of the car window and watched the rain-slicked, wind-blown north coast landscape reel by. "How," I asked myself, crying, "can a child who cannot handle labor, handle life on planet earth?"

Once in the hospital, they hooked me up to the monitor and we waited. I had a few weak Braxton-Hicks contractions, but we were able to stimulate some stronger contractions by rubbing my breasts. The baby's heart rate went up during each one, which was good news; the baby's score was acceptable. We saw another doctor before heading home. He checked my dates again and examined me; my cervix was soft, but not effaced.

That night at 12:30 a.m., I woke up with pains five minutes apart. We were so thrilled, so happy, so excited, so *ready*. The storm was abating amid great displays of lightning; our neighbor drove us the forty-minute journey to the home of Alison, another midwife who had lovingly come to our aid. We all had our minds set against a hospital birth, believing all was well. A compromise was reached when Alison offered her home, which was relatively close to town, for me to labor in and, providing my waters were clear, deliver in. (Waters stained with meconium can indicate fetal distress.)

Slowly, steadily, somewhat like a roller coaster, my rushes commenced. I was feeling the pain that no one had been able to explain, but I tried to maintain my sense of humor. Walking, walking, walking into the moonlit night, gravity doing its work while we did ours: breathe, breathe, breathe, cleansing breath. Mary, Becca and Lorraine kept tabs on the baby, listening, feeling, telling me how well I was doing. "Getting closer, doing fine." I was in and out of the hot bath more than once, which gave me a chance to relax. I found it difficult to keep my eyes open or do much moving around once my labor got more intense. I slept a little between contractions. The ladies, all eight of them, would get me up and make me walk. Eventually Mary told me she was going to break my waters. There was a flurry of activity as a car was prepared in the event that my waters were stained, and we would have to go to the hospital.

My waters were stained, though just faintly. We all said, "What are we going to do?" In spite of our plans, I was propped up on the couch and I pushed. We all worked together. "Push, blow, blow, blow, push on!" It felt so intense I thought Mary had her hand in my anus. She massaged my perineum with olive oil and the baby slipped out at 9:00 a.m. She started breathing, gave a squack or two and immediately took my breast. One ripe cherry falling to earth. Six and a half pounds and she didn't look overdue. My placenta, healthy and whole, came with a push on the following contraction.

I was so elated, so high, so ready to get on with life and be done with the waiting. It was a sunny day; the carrot juice was soothing my head and nerves. We said goodbye to the midwives as they took off for other places, and I was finally able to rest—the best gift of all for a new momma.

*Jolynn and her daughter Jasmine find joy in a fulfilling family life and working on the land. Music, horseback riding and other creative releases are their pleasures. Jolynn teaches music to elementary school children.*

# In a Cabin In the Woods

by Gail Stebbins

Alicia Laurel's birth was a magical event for me and her father Malcolm. He was the only person present at her birth; he gave me support and helped to deliver her. He says all he did was catch the baby; I know the truth—he gave me courage and strength, light and warmth.

Alicia was born almost two weeks after her due date. Day after day we would wait and wonder, Will this be the day? Finally one morning I woke at 2:18 and my water had broken. I could feel it trickling down my leg inside my sweatpants. I immediately woke Malcolm and told him. He got excited and started preparing for the birth. He put the water on the stove to boil and the plastic sheet on the bed; then he went to the car to call the midwives, Lorraine and Mary, on the CB but was unable to reach them. When he came back into the cabin, I was having a strong contraction. He stayed with me until the contraction was over and then went back to the car to call again but still couldn't reach anyone, not even the other people with whom we had arranged to relay messages.

My contractions continued to be strong and hard. I went outside to pee, or so I thought, but then felt like I needed to have the biggest bowel movement in the world. I screamed and couldn't stand up. I looked up at the sky and noticed an almost full moon, and the dog across the river started to howl. Malcolm helped me walk back to the cabin. We knelt on the bed together with our arms around each other, hugging and kissing spontaneously. It seemed like everything was going so fast. I was happy, although there were moments when I thought I wouldn't be able to go through with it. But a little voice inside gave me confidence and told me to be open and loving, to stay relaxed, and to just keep opening up.

Malcolm said he would go the neighbors to use their phone when the contraction I was having was over. The neighbors weren't too far away, but I was afraid and didn't want to be left alone, so I asked him not to leave. He said, "OK, I'll stay. Now, breathe."

I told him, "I don't remember how!"

He said, "Pant, pant, blow."

I did that and said, "Now what?"

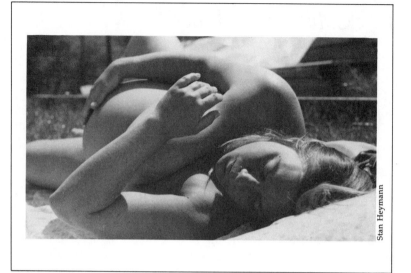

Stan Heymann

He said, "Breathe again."

It was 3:00 a.m., forty minutes after my water had broken. I was kneeling on our bed, on my hands and knees, pushing, when the baby squirted out into Malcolm's hands as I watched between my legs. He said, "It's a girl and she's perfect!" I rolled over onto my back, and he placed her wet little body on my chest. At first we just lay there looking at each other, then we figured out how to nurse. Malcolm clamped the cord and cut it about an hour later. I squinched my eyes and held my breath thinking it might hurt Alicia or me. Of course we didn't feel a thing except a slight loss and a little fear of separation. From that moment on, the three of us have been more together than ever.

Lorraine and Mary felt slightly left out when they arrived at 6:00 a.m. They came into our dark little cabin and checked me to be sure there had been no problems with the delivery. I had only a slight tear. They delivered the placenta (which Malcolm and I hadn't known how to do) and cleaned Alicia and me up. Lorraine and Mary made several visits after the birth to be sure we were doing fine, and they became good friends of our family. Their role as teachers and midwives, as well as friends, was truly valuable.

*Gail and her husband have been working to build their home and barn which will be powered by wind, water and solar electricity. They love animals, and Gail enjoys gardening, singing, dancing and family life.*

# Babes for a Greybeard and a Young Lady

by Ruth Harper

My husband Daniel bravely decided to have a second family with me. As he is thirty-one years my senior and has children older than I, it was a big decision. He sat in the waiting room for the births of his first two offspring; for his second family, he assisted at the births. He says there is no comparison.

A Russian Grand Duchess and a Maine seaport inspired the names of our two babes. Daniel and I had independently thought, long before we met, that if we ever had a little girl we'd name her Anastasia. It was too much of a coincidence to ignore. Camden is the Maine seaport where we started our relationship and we felt that the event should be remembered in our son's name.

❦     ❦     ❦

Anastasia, our first baby, was born in the local hospital after a four-hour labor. We decided on a hospital birth as I was very comfortable with the setting, having worked there for two and a half years. Never having given birth, I felt better in a hospital in case the baby needed immediate care.

I lost my mucus plug five days before I went into labor. For three days I had regular Braxton-Hicks contractions and when Lorraine, my midwife, checked my progress, I was 1-2 centimeters dilated. Lorraine stayed that night, but when there was no change by the next morning, she left, encouraging me to be as active as possible all day. My due date was still two weeks away.

I followed her advice, ate lightly, and had a busy and tense day of waiting. When Lorraine called that evening, it seemed as if our little babe wasn't quite ready. Lorraine said to get back on a regular diet and not to worry; I probably wouldn't have the baby for days.

I went to bed shortly after eating a hearty meal, feeling slightly depressed at my lack of progress. After a few hours of sleep, I awoke suddenly, not knowing exactly what was happening. I was very wet—had my water broken? After a few minutes I was gripped by overpowering contractions accompanied by diarrhea, nausea and some bleeding. Dan got out the flow chart for what to expect in a normal labor and starting at the top with 1-2 centimeters, he quickly dropped to the bottom of the list with 8-10 centimeter dilation and transition. Panic! He contacted Lorraine through a friend with a CB radio —she was on her way.

With each of the contractions, which were coming two to three minutes apart, I would call Dan, who was running around getting things together. He would come into the bathroom, hold my hand and help me through it. It was amazing how his direct look encouraged me. I was only comfortable sitting on the toilet; I was there when Lorraine arrived a half hour later. Her presence had a very calming effect on me. When she checked me, I was almost completely dilated.

"Don't you need to push?" asked Lorraine.

"Now that you mention it . . . " I replied with the next contraction.

"Don't!" said Lorraine.

We had a *very* brief discussion as to whether or not to go to the hospital and decided to go ahead as planned. Dan warmed up our VW Bug while I threw on an odd array of clothes. Lorraine and I crawled into the back seat and off we went. The drive seemed to go on forever even though it was only two and a half miles. Lorraine shined a flashlight on her face so I could watch her and blow, not push, with each contraction.

We arrived at the hospital shortly after 1:00 a.m., only two hours after my labor had started. As I had prearranged, I was allowed to use a regular private room rather than the labor and delivery room for my birth. When Dr. Bill arrived, shortly after we did, he checked me and told me to go ahead and push. Bill and Lorraine sat on the end of the bed, and as a team, coached me; Dan stayed by my side giving me lots of support. Pushing was a very hard concept for me to grasp. It wasn't until the end of each contraction that I would start to push correctly.

As the baby's head crowned both of us were told to touch her head. What a thrill! That gave me more encouragement than any words could have. I had breaks between contractions, some lasting as long as ten minutes. I enjoyed those rest periods as there was no discomfort, and I wasn't tired since my labor had been so short. We all joked and talked during these recesses, and I had time to think about becoming a momma soon.

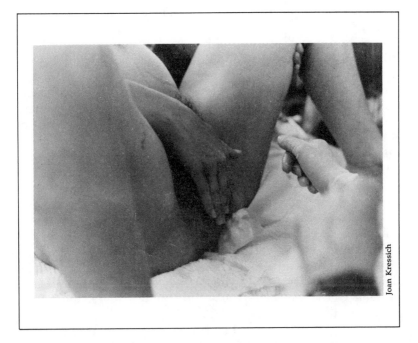

Joan Kressich

The last few pushes burned. The harder I pushed the more it burned, but I knew those hard pushes would get her out sooner. Bill and Lorraine worked well together. When the baby was born, they checked her—she was perfect. She was placed on my now-flat tummy. Bill gave Dan the scissors to cut her cord. Tears were in all our eyes as we "oohed" and "aahed" at our accomplishment.

Our baby Anastasia was beautiful at birth, but became more so as the day broke. It was truly fabulous to watch her face unfold like a flower during those first few hours. I never tired of looking at our babe and was amazed to the point of tears at what we had done.

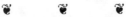

We were overjoyed when, eleven months later, we found I was pregnant with our second baby. We had wanted another child and had planned on having them close together.

As with Anastasia, I had very bad morning sickness with a weight loss of more than twenty pounds and some unusual bleeding. I had to spend a lot of time resting quietly. I was nursing Anastasia and was told to stop nursing and not to pick up anything over ten pounds—not easy advice to follow with an eleven-month-old baby.

I believed that Anastasia and her new sibling would have little rivalry and a good relationship if I continued nursing until Anastasia weaned herself; however, it was not easy. My milk disappeared by the third month and towards the end of my pregnancy my nipples got very sore. No matter how much I discouraged her, Anastasia never gave up—a sign to me that she still needed to nurse. As my time drew nearer, I had so little patience with Anastasia that I questioned my ability to keep my sanity with two children.

We decided to have the second baby at home. We were well prepared: We bought a sofa bed for downstairs, had backup lighting in case of an electrical failure, and went through emergency childbirth procedures with Lorraine.

Dan started his paternity leave three weeks before my due date. I was frustrated and tired trying to organize everything while taking care of Anastasia. Having Dan around really helped, and we managed to clean the house thoroughly and get the baby's clothes ready.

Five days after Dan started his leave, I woke with a stitch in my side, a constant Braxton-Hicks contraction and a rotten feeling all over. I stopped at the Clinic to ask if what I was feeling meant anything and I was told I had been doing too much and not to worry; they didn't think it was necessary to examine me. By late afternoon I felt as if I was starting to have some regular contractions. We sterilized the birthing packs, and I began timing the contractions, realizing I had to sit down and breathe with them. Maybe this was the real thing.

Lorraine had told me that I wouldn't go into labor until I felt ready. She also said that women usually don't go into hard labor until their other children are taken care of. Both theories were true for me: I was mentally prepared as the house was clean and the birthing supplies were ready, and I had only a few contractions that required my full attention before we settled Anastasia for the night.

I called Lorraine at 7:00 p.m. to tell her what was happening. She said she didn't think it was a false alarm and that she would come over in a couple of hours unless we called her again.

By 8:30 p.m. my contractions were coming every five to seven minutes. Since I was still fairly comfortable I decided to go upstairs to spend some time in our family bed with Anastasia. I remember thinking that the next time I saw her there would be two children, and our relationship would be very different. I kissed her "good-bye," not realizing how different it would be.

When Lorraine arrived I came back downstairs. She checked my progress and found I was 6-7 centimeters dilated; she thought I would have the baby before midnight. Daniel and Lorraine readied the house as I moved quietly around having contractions. By 10:30 p.m., when Kathleen arrived, the labor had not picked up remarkably. I took a shower and went without clothes; had I been in the hospital, I would not have been as comfortable. Daniel took a picture for posterity.

The labor progressed more slowly than Lorraine had predicted, but by 1:00 a.m. I could feel the change as the baby entered the birth canal. I had a hard time keeping it together after that. The burning sensation started sooner than it had with Anastasia and I remember thinking, I want this over *soon*. I tried all sorts of positions, but it went very slowly.

At about 1:30 a.m. I had an unusually heavy show of blood. The midwives weren't sure of its exact cause, but the baby was doing fine. They asked me to try squatting, but after just a few contractions I wanted to get back into bed. No position was comfortable, and I was holding back knowing how much the burning sensation hurt, but realizing the harder I pushed the sooner it would be over.

We had discussed with the midwives what to do with Anastasia during the birth. They felt that older siblings take to the new baby much better if they are present at the birth. We decided to wake Anastasia just as the baby was crowning, giving me most of my labor without her so I could concentrate. When Daniel brought her down, she cried a little but then sat and quietly watched. Still half asleep, she was in the perfect frame of mind to watch without needing too much attention.

Daniel wanted to help deliver the baby instead of merely staying by my side. I was somewhat concerned because I thought I would feel better with him beside me, but everyone at the birth gave so much support that his role as "catcher" worked out very well. Kathleen and Daniel exchanged places after Anastasia was settled, and we moved into the final phase. I was encouraged to touch the baby's head, giving me that burst of energy needed to get the baby out. Finally there was a tangible conclusion to a painful experience.

As the head appeared, Lorraine exclaimed that the baby was

"sunny side up," an unusual position which explained the pro-longed time in the birth canal and the burning. Lorraine suctioned the babe's nose and mouth; then I gave a last push and the body came out. When I asked Lorraine if it was a girl or boy, she insisted that Daniel tell me. He looked and said, "I'm not sure, but I think it's a boy."

"Are you sure?" I asked, as we had wanted a girl.

"It's got balls, honey!" Kathleen said.

Lorraine assured me it was true and put the little lad up on my tummy. Daniel later said he thought he was looking at the umbilical cord, hence the confusion. We had only thought of having a girl, so changing was hard. It took us a few weeks to adjust, but now I wouldn't change the way it turned out for anything.

After holding and nursing Camden, Lorraine took him while Kathleen helped me deliver the placenta. It was split right down the middle. Lorraine had never seen anything like it and thought that the split might have caused the bleeding prior to the birth.

I really enjoyed the homebirth. Not being separated from the new baby and relaxing at home with my whole family were wonderful and I felt completely safe having two competent midwives in attendance. Anastasia seemed genuinely pleased and kept kissing her new brother; she was not at all upset by the birth. We had an ideal situation, and I hope that if we have any more children we can duplicate it.

*Ruth, Dan and their two children have moved to the coast of Maine where they own and operate a bed and breakfast inn. Ruth writes that her family and the inn are her priorities now but that she hopes to return to work in the medical field someday.*

# Two Births: Logan and Ana Rose

by Linda Walter

At the age of twenty, unmarried and unsettled, I was very unsure of what to do when I found myself pregnant. After the initial shock passed, Christopher and I decided we'd keep the baby and have it by natural childbirth. We toured a San Francisco hospital and were quite impressed by its alternative birth center. The birthing rooms were comfortably furnished and the births were attended by Certified Nurse-Midwives. Physicians were just a few rooms away in case they were needed. At that time I wasn't confident about my ability to give birth without a doctor nearby, and since the apartment we had just moved into didn't seem much like home, we thought the birth center would be the best place to have the baby.

Pregnancy gave me few physical problems—I did lots of walking. Chris and I took Lamaze classes, and I read books on birth and pregnancy. *Birth Without Violence* by Frédérick Leboyer made a strong impression on me, and I began to feel more sure of myself and my desire for a non-violent birth as the nine months of preparation passed.

One morning I woke up, got out of bed and found water streaming down my legs. The water bag had burst. I called the hospital and started getting things ready. Chris and I hopped on the bus to do some last-minute errands. I was unaware that I would continue to produce more and more water; much of the sacred fluid was sprinkled on the streets of San Francisco.

When we arrived at the hospital early the next day, labor hadn't started yet. It had been nearly twenty-four hours since the water had broken. Chris and I tried various things to start labor. I drank some herb teas a friend brought, even subjected myself to an enema, but nothing happened. According to hospital rules, twenty-four hours with broken water was too long. I was moved out of the birth center into a white-walled labor room, and given Pitocin from an IV. A very businesslike clinic physician was on duty, and she offered little sympathy. The nurses kept increasing the dose of Pitocin but still nothing happened. After a couple of hours and a lot of Pitocin, I started experiencing frequent painful

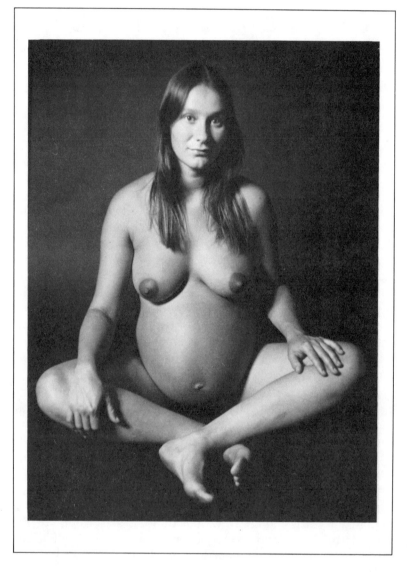

contractions. The monitor I was hooked up to showed the baby's heart rate slowing down dangerously with each contraction. The impersonal physician came in and said I might need a cesarean section. Fifteen minutes later, after I was abruptly shaved, catheterized and wheeled to the operating room, Logan was pulled out into the world. He was screaming and would not stop.

Chris was not allowed to go in the operating room or even to peek in the window, but he did get to hold our son soon after he was born. Logan weighed eight pounds, eleven ounces and barely fit through the "bikini cut" hole the surgeon had made. She had wanted to do a long vertical incision, but Chris persuaded her not to, telling her that I liked to do belly dancing. I myself had been too frightened and confused to question anything the hospital staff did or said.

Two hours after the birth I emerged from a drug-induced fog and was wheeled to see my husband and son. The attendant wheeled Logan out of the nursery to meet me, and when I saw him for the first time, our eyes locked and he stopped screaming. He knew me, and I knew him; in spite of a bad start, a beautiful relationship was just beginning.

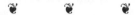

When I became pregnant again a year later, I was anxious not to repeat any of the mistakes I had made the first time. I wanted to avoid hospitals, but midwives in San Francisco, Northern California and Oregon were all unwilling to attempt a homebirth for a previously c-sectioned woman. Doctors in different cities told me they couldn't guarantee even a trial labor. I was a high-risk case now, they said, and my uterus could rupture. In spite of this, Chris, Logan and I moved to the country, hoping that healthier living would help me have a more successful labor and delivery.

The best thing that happened to me during my pregnancy was meeting the midwives at the Clinic, a couple hours' drive from where we lived. They were sympathetic, caring women, unlike the doctor who had delivered Logan. They worked closely with a country doctor who said he'd let me try a vaginal birth if the hospital could get three doctors to stand by in case emergency surgery became necessary.

The nine months passed, and after a night of little sleep I began to notice twinges in my belly that were occuring regularly. By noon I knew it was real labor, and I was ecstatic because I had never experienced natural contractions before. A phone call to the hospital informed us that Dr. Bill was out of town, but the midwives said they'd try to set something up for us elsewhere.

We started the long, winding drive to the highway. Rain was pouring down and thunder boomed in the distance. There was a lot of water on the road, so we took it slowly. We had a copy of the police and firemen's manual, *Emergency Childbirth*, by Gregory White, with us in the van, along with pillows, blankets, water and sterile gloves. The midwives had told us that if the baby was coming fast there would probably be no complications.

We stopped at a pay phone on the highway to call the midwives. They told us to drive north to a larger city where a doctor they knew had agreed to do our birth for us. We began driving down a road that was totally flooded out, jumpstarted a stalled car, and then went north by another route.

That evening, we met for the first time the doctor who was to deliver our baby. To our surprise he wore his hair in a ponytail like Chris and we really liked him. He asked us some questions about my pregnancy and the cesarean I'd had and said he'd be glad to let me try a vaginal birth. We later learned that he was new at the hospital and was bending some established rules to do this.

Chris and I put on robes, and we walked to and from the bathroom and all around the hospital for hours. I began to feel discouraged because labor was starting to hurt a lot, but I was making no real progress; I was stuck at 3 centimeters for at least five hours. I had some bleeding, and since I didn't know how much to expect, I was afraid they might strap me down and roll me off to surgery again. The contractions got stronger, and I began feeling so much residual pain from my previous birth that I wished they would do a cesarean to get it over with.

Around 2:00 a.m., a loud clap of thunder shook the hospital. The doctor came in to check my dilation and found I was finally starting to open up. Labor was much easier after that. Chris pushed on my back during the contractions, which helped a great deal. He also kept in touch with the midwives by telephone, and they told him encouraging things to say to me. I began to feel much more positive as the time neared to go to the delivery room.

I let the doctor put a glucose IV in my arm even though my last birth experience had made me afraid of IV's. I also had to put my feet in stirrups, but I compromised. The nurses wanted to shave me, but the doctor said, "You don't really need to do that, do you? Just wash her." Chris put his arms around me from behind, lifted up my torso and pushed with me. The water bag burst and splashed on everyone. A few more good pushes and I could see the baby's head emerge. The doctor held her by the shoulders, and she slid right out. They laid the baby on my chest with the cord still attached. Ana Rose looked so small, weighing only seven pounds, and lay very peacefully and quietly as I nursed her on the delivery table.

The next day when I was resting in my hospital room, one of the nurses who had helped with Ana's birth came to visit me. She said that it was the first time a woman with a previous c-section had given birth vaginally in that hospital and that she was very glad to have been there. So, Ana Rose had made a little history coming into the world. More significantly to me, her birth restored my confidence in myself and in my body's ability to function naturally. I am now certain that women have the power within their bodies to give birth in a natural way. But it is necessary to choose people and methods that go along with, rather than against, these natural energies of childbirth. Contrary to my expectations, I found that even a hospital birth could be a positive experience.

*Linda and her two children live in a valley near a river. In addition to gardening, raising animals and working on her homestead, she enjoys sewing, hiking and volleyball.*

# This Child Abram
by Mick Burkholder


To his parents' delight,
this child Abram
born on a whispery subtle night . . .

Clouds huddled close to the earth ~
The wind stopped holding its breath ~
Oaks . . . Firs . . .
and all the gathering trees
bend close to see,
stirring not a leaf or needle.

From deep inside
he moved to the rhythm of mystery.
Pulled by lunar mother,
surrounded by his angelic earth mother.
Loving attendants ~
~ Father ~ Midwife ~ earth sister
harmonizing the primal energy . . .

The long moment extends
as the crest of the head appears,
dips back . . . time after time . . .
Crowning ~ pushing ~ blowing ~ burning . . .
Oh help, it burns so bad!
One more, just one more.
Push! Oh my! Look at the size of his head.
Sit back mama, take it easy for a moment . . .
The pink head lies quite still
as mucus is sucked from nose and mouth,
and we wait . . .

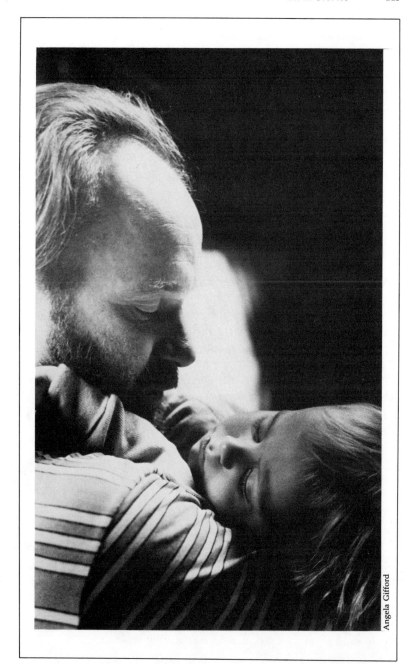

Angela Gifford

Standing in winter brown coats, the deer,
with long erect ears, gaze,
large round compassionate eyes
in absolute stillness . . .
One more push!
And the shoulders slide
past overstretched skin.

Little Abram sings wha a a a . . .
And the world breathes a joyous sweet breath,
the wind stirs, the trees bow,
as tears of gladness flow.

*After working in the Peace Corps for two years and visiting East Asian countries, Mick discovered that the rural way of living suited his disposition. He learned to build and garden, and develop the hundreds of skills that mountain dwellers use in daily life. He says, "My lovely Angela and darling children are now the fullest part of this adventure which leads me in search of the true values that nurture all life. As I travel this road of pitfalls, finding my way with family and friends, I seek for the pure gold of patience and understanding."*

# New Dimensions

by Angela Gifford

---

I believe that each time a woman gives birth there is something new to be learned from the experience. There is always a certain amount of work to be done which can manifest itself in any number of ways. My last birth was so wonderfully smooth and easy that I asked myself, Where were the lessons? Where was the work? Ah hah! For me it was the pregnancy—the physical strain, the wondering, the intense emotional decisions and the waiting—that was my work.

I knew from the beginning that there was something different about this pregnancy. My initial reaction to these feelings was that maybe something was wrong. I feared the possibility of a miscarriage or an abnormal baby. These fears seemed to dissipate after the first months, and I knew it was a healthy pregnancy. Still there was something unique about it, something I had yet to discover.

❦        ❦        ❦

The physical demand on my body was incredible. I was working as a cook at a small alternative school and had a three-year-old son to look after. The first month passed and morning sickness set in. I tried to ignore it although working in a kitchen with a nauseous stomach wasn't easy. I forced protein drinks and carrot juice down just to stay on my feet. My body's nutritional demands were so great that I could go no more than an hour without food. This surprised me—I couldn't believe that my body was burning this food-energy so quickly. It was almost ridiculous at times. I would feel a light-headed sensation which meant I had minutes to get something down, or I would pass out.

By the third month I was bulging out of my pants. I began wondering why this was happening so quickly. I felt a constant tightening in my uterus and could actually feel it stretching. I asked Kathleen, one of my midwives, to measure my belly several times during the first few months. She always did so with a smile and responded to my concern in her usual reassuring way, "With second pregnancies you tend to get big much sooner." I talked to other second-time mothers who confirmed this—a few had felt so big that they were sure they were carrying twins, only to find one healthy baby. My curiosity wavered back and forth. One part of me was convinced that I was nurturing two babies, yet the outward signs and opinions were just as certain that there was only one. I accepted my ever-growing belly with the attitude, Time will tell.

During my fifth month I was so big that people began to ask if my baby was due soon. I could only laugh. By the sixth month the question was rephrased, "Is it any time now?" I would smile and reply, "Any time in the next three months."

Here I was, only six months along, and I was feeling the discomforts that most women feel in their ninth month. I could no longer lie on my back because the weight of my belly would cut off my oxygen and I'd become faint. It was difficult to find a comfortable position when I slept.

As time went on, I became more certain that there must be two babies, and my mission was to find just one person who agreed with me. In my many discussions with Mick, my husband, I came close to convincing him, yet the mere thought of twins was a bit overwhelming for him to accept. We went to see our good friend and midwife Lily in hopes of finding a more definite answer. In earlier visits she had said that she intuitively felt that there was just one big baby with a lot of water. During this visit, however, I noticed a glimmer of doubt cross her face when she found two heartbeats in different parts of my belly. But amazingly, the heartbeats were synchronized, which is unusual. When I went to the Clinic for my seven-month exam, the midwives also heard heartbeats in two locations, but again they were synchronized. No one was willing to say that I was carrying twins because the sound of the heartbeat can bounce off the wall of the uterus and be heard in different places. Dr. Bill suggested that I have a sonogram the following week. I gladly agreed. The day finally came and all the way into town Mick and I would look at each other and smile, him saying, "There's just one," and me replying, "There's two."

After all the waiting and wondering, in just one minute of scanning my belly the radiologist turned off the machine and said quite seriously, "There's *at least* two in there!" I had known already, yet hearing those words made a great impact. Tears welled up in my eyes as I looked over at Mick and Lily, who were bracing themselves against one another, their mouths gaping open.

The radiologist then did a very thorough scan of both babies. I was amazed at the amount of information gathered, the most significant being their approximate weights and positions: Twin A, head down and presenting first, weighed four pounds. Twin B, breech, weighed three and a half pounds. He was also fairly certain in identifying their sexes. Twin A was a boy, Twin B, a girl. This delighted us—one of each which meant they were fraternal.

With this discovery came much joy and excitement, yet our simple decision to have a homebirth was now more complicated. I knew, having had my first child at home, that for me it was the ideal place to be, but I was afraid that I would not be able to find anyone to support such a decision. I also knew that an even greater responsibility would be placed on me. Was I willing to accept this? In sharing these feelings with Mick, I was surprised to find that he also felt most comfortable with a homebirth assuming there were no complications. Lily also felt confident with a home delivery. I was overjoyed for I knew that together we would find the strength that was necessary.

There was so much preparation to be done. We began gathering as much information on twin deliveries as we could. My first challenge was to keep the babies inside until they were big and healthy. Twins tend to be born prematurely, which creates several complications. In the book *Having Twins* by Elizabeth Noble, I read that good nutrition is the key for a healthy delivery, and I began eating 3000-4000 calories a day and increased my vitamin supplements. Another major consideration was that the second baby was in a breech position. Lily had delivered one breech baby and felt confident and even excited with this new opportunity. Together we researched and studied breech delivery techniques.

My due date was December 22. By mid-November my body began showing signs of readiness. During one of my prenatal exams, Lorraine decided to check my cervix, which she normally would not have done that early. I remember looking down at her and seeing her smile fade to a look of concern. She said that my cervix was softening and I was about 1 centimeter dilated. Generally with these signs, labor can begin at any time. I was so taken aback by this that I cried. How could I have felt so strong, then suddenly feel so helpless? She suggested that I rest and keep to a minimal amount of activity. We made an agreement that if the babies were to come before December 1, I would go to the hospital to have them.

I began to get very depressed lying around the house like an invalid, worrying that labor might happen at any time. This went on for about a week. Then I came across an article on bedrest which said that this method of preventing labor is no longer suggested because the psychological impact of waiting can actually cause women to go into labor. I had also become very weak from lack of exercise and knew that I was in no condition to give birth. This was a turning point in my pregnancy. I understood the demands on my body and knew what felt right for me. I decided to take control of my situation instead of letting it control me. With a positive attitude and plenty of food I was going to hold the babies comfortably inside until they were ready.

With great anticipation, December 1 finally arrived. I was relieved and delighted. We had overcome our first obstacle, and the babies were now big enough to be born at home.

My sister Sara arrived at the end of the week. She planned to be at the birth. My confidence soared. Sara's strength and gentleness have always touched me in a special way. We went walking every day. I felt like a ninety-year-old woman walking on glass. "Tighter," I'd say as she cinched the sash that was supporting my belly, and off we'd go, a mile on a country road.

One morning I awoke with a slight pain in my side. As I got up and moved around it became worse. I had felt this before. The babies, in struggling for more room, would get an elbow or a knee stuck deep in my side. I would get into different positions and try to nudge them out. With perseverance, it always worked. This particular time I could see Twin B's body turned sideways digging deep into my side. I told her that I knew she was trying to turn head down, but it was too late and there was simply *no* room for such a maneuver. All day I lay on the couch pleading with her, crying a bit and wondering how long it would go on. By evening she let up, and I was grateful. The following day I went to the Clinic for my weekly exam. As Lily palpated my belly she seemed puzzled and went to get Lorraine for a second opinion. Sure enough, Twin B was now head down. The wonders of nature amazed us all.

Two weeks from my due date, I was beginning to catch a second wind. I knew it would happen sooner or later. My body began to adjust to the extra sixty-five pounds and the awkwardness of a forty-five-inch waistline (all in front). The days passed slowly, filled with the spirit of the Christmas season. It was wonderful to spend this time with my little boy Abram, for I knew that all too soon there would barely be enough time for him.

Phone calls came daily from friends and relatives wondering if the babies had arrived yet. My father, even though he was first on the list to be called, phoned at least every other day with his wondering and overly anxious concerns. It got to the point that when we heard the phone ring, Sara and I would look at one another and volunteer Mick to answer it. My due date, December 22, arrived. It was a rather uneventful day. Who would have guessed when I rushed to do Christmas shopping in November that I'd be looking for things to keep me busy during December.

Christmas Eve came and the mood was one of silent anticipation: Mick, Sara and I wondering if I was going to give birth on Christmas day; Abram wondering if Santa Claus was really coming that night.

Sara and I were up until about 1:00 a.m. Shortly after I had gone to sleep I was awakened by some fairly strong contractions. They seemed to be regular at two-minute intervals. This must be it, I thought. Mick got up and called Lily at 2:00 a.m. As soon as Mick talked to her, the contractions stopped. I couldn't believe it! Lily asked a few questions and sensed that it wasn't really happening yet. She told Mick to call back if I showed any other signs. I slept all night.

Morning arrived—this was Abram's Christmas. It was quiet and warm with love. He was the child and his eyes sparkled with excitement.

Christmas was over and the waiting began to wear on me. Concerns grew heavy. Dr. Bill commented, "Overdue twins—I've never heard of such a thing!"

One day while sunning my belly, I picked up a case of poison oak from petting my cat. It came out all over my huge belly. It was one of the most offensive things that could have happened. It spread to my thighs. I was miserable. The thought of laboring in such a condition was out of the question. I sat for hours in baths of herbal remedies, my only relief.

Felicia, another sister, arrived; she offered great moral support. I needed this support far more for the case of poison oak than for labor. My energy focused solely on clearing it up; I could think of nothing else. By the end of the week it showed some signs of healing. Thank goodness.

We went to a New Year's Eve party. I sat quietly most of the evening, watching Sara and Mick dance to Greek music.

Felicia had to return home to her family, and we were all disappointed that she had to go. My courage was beginning to melt, yet I had a strong sense that everything was fine, and I trusted the babies to come when they were ready. My cervix had been dilating for two months and at my last prenatal exam I was 5 centimeters.

Mick and Lily began to get concerned. One evening, I overheard them talking on the phone about calling the hospital simply to ask them what they thought about it. I don't know why I was so sensitive about this, but I felt like I was being abandoned. I was hurt that they didn't trust my intuitions.

Mick and I went on a long walk in the misty rain. We discussed our feelings and concerns. There were tears and long embraces. We returned home to a quiet house. It felt good to reconnect with one another.

❦          ❦          ❦

Early the next morning I was awakened by a sharp blow to my belly—it felt as though someone had punched me. I gasped as I sat up abruptly. What was that? I then realized that the blow had come from within and at that moment I felt water pouring out of me. This was it, it was finally happening. I knew that things would go quickly, for I had been 5 centimeters dilated the day before. We woke Sara, and Mick called the midwives, Lily, Kathleen and Lorraine—they were on their way. I sat downstairs alone while Sara and Mick made preparations. I felt my body surge with contractions. I took slow deep breaths. I talked to the babies, letting them know that I was with them and that we were going to work together and not be afraid.

When the midwives arrived half an hour later, I was in transition. The contractions were very intense, but with new excitement and concentration I was able to work with them. Visualizing my cervix softening and opening, I seemed to transcend the pain.

I decided it was time to go upstairs while I could still get around. The room was cozy and warm with candles burning. Abram was curled up in his bed next to ours, asleep.

Friends arrived and came upstairs to greet me. Although I seemed lost in contractions, I was very aware of the details surrounding me. I noticed the camera flashing my picture and commented, "Save it for the babies." At one point I looked around the room, and seeing all the friendly faces filled with concern I thought a bit of comic relief was necessary, so I conjured up a sense of humor.

The contractions continued to grow stronger, and still I main-

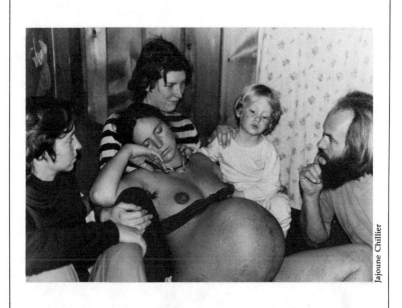

Jajoune Chillier

tained a self-control which surprised even me. Lily checked me and I was fully dilated. I did not feel a strong urge to push but gave a few practice pushes to get a feel for it. I was sitting on the bed leaning back against Kathleen. I felt a sharp digging pain—Twin B was being pushed over to the side to make room for Twin A. It was quite painful. Finally I shifted my weight to the other side and found relief. I remember wondering how the baby felt being pushed to the side.

Abram soon woke up to a room filled with friends, and with sheer delight announced, "The babies! The babies are coming!" He snuggled up next to me with wide eyes and was wonderful throughout the births.

It was difficult pushing while on the bed. I stood through a few contractions and then sat down on a toilet-like seat. This felt very solid, yet was open on my bottom. The air space beneath me made the difference. Twin A required a lot of pushing. With my first birth I had pushed for three hours, and I expected the same with this baby, although he came more quickly. I pushed when I felt like it, taking little breaks in between and not expending all my energy, for in the back of my mind I knew there would be a lot more work in delivering yet another baby. The midwives sat beside me watching with sweet, reassuring eyes. I would tell them what I was feeling, and that was all they needed to know for the moment.

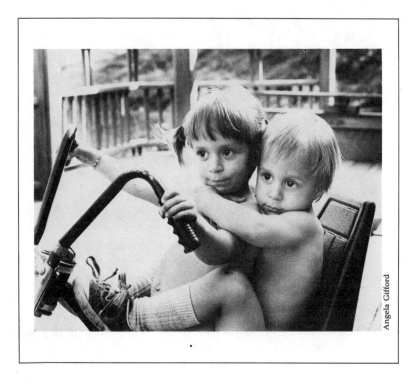

Angela Gifford

I felt the head move down as I pushed and slip back up when I stopped. It was getting close and starting to burn. I knew it was time to get back onto the bed. With a few more pushes I reached down and felt a soft wet head emerging. Another push and there he was, Miko Hans, born into Mick's loving hands at 5:50 a.m. He was beautiful and made a couple of little sounds to say hello. I held him for a moment while the cord was cut, then passed him to his papa. He lay in Mick's lap, silent, looking around with wide eyes, waiting patiently for his sister to arrive.

The contractions stopped, and it was nice to relax for a moment. My cervix went back to 8 centimeters. I stood up and moved around, which helped stimulate contractions. Twin B was high in the pelvis. Lily tried to rupture the membrane. I gave a few pushes.

I had a strong sense of time and knew its importance even though there was no outside pressure on me. The midwives remained confident, and they had faith in my intuition and I in theirs. This was a wonderful feeling and gave me strength. I knew this baby would come much quicker, and with just a few pushes I felt great pressure in my vagina. I thought, Could this be the head already? Gee, that was easy. I told the midwives that it felt like the head was crowning, and walked to the bed holding it with my hand, just in case. To everyone's disappointment what I thought was the head was a bulging sack of water. Lily broke it and said the baby was still very high up. Somewhat discouraged, I returned to the seat and began pushing with a strength I must have gathered from the universe. Time passing, I pushed with great determination. After a few very intense pushes, the head moved down quickly. I felt her starting to crown, and I made it back to the bed. Another good push and the head was out. Lily suctioned her a little and she cried. I reached down and felt her warmth. Her hand was by her face. With a little push, there she was, my daughter, Dia Hana, born at 6:49 a.m. Two babies! The wonder of it all! I brought them to my breast, and they both nursed. What a sensation.

Twenty minutes passed, and I got up to deliver the placenta. It came right away, followed by a gush of blood. The midwives acted quickly by giving me several herbal tinctures for hemorrhage and massaging the uterus while the babies sucked. The bleeding was under control, but I was experiencing mild shock. They watched me carefully, and I remained lying down. I had put all responsibility into their hands, for what really mattered to me now were my two beautiful healthy babies that I snuggled in each arm.

My body recovered fairly quickly from the shock. I watched Lily bundle each baby in a receiving blanket and place them on her scale. Miko weighed eight pounds, one ounce; Dia, seven pounds, five ounces. That was impressive!

I would stare at them for hours in awe that there were really two of them. Overflowing with love and joy, I was so proud of myself for being a mother.

*After graduating from Chico State University with a degree in child development, Angela began her career in the field as a fulltime mother with her first son Abram. Six years later, when the twins were two years old, she returned to work as a teacher at a Montessori preschool. Angela says she enjoys gardening, photography, running, family walks and starry nights.*

# Aurianna Miranda and Micah David

by Mary Bendle

---

It was four weeks until our first baby was due. One day my husband Michael and I sat rubbing my belly saying, "You can come out now, little baby. We want to see you and play with you." To our surprise my water broke during the night. This being our first pregnancy, we didn't know how labor would progress, so we decided to get some more sleep. The next morning, we went to my prenatal checkup.

The doctor told us my cervix hadn't begun to thin out, and that with broken waters it wasn't a good idea to wait too long for labor to start because of the chance of infection. After thirty hours and no contractions, the only alternative was induction. Although we had hoped for a homebirth, we packed our bags and with our midwife, Lily, we headed for the hospital.

Pitocin induction was a hard way to go. I was confined to bed with a fetal heart monitor and an IV that made it almost impossible for me to move around. I got the shakes, vomited and begged for drugs. The only security and comfort I felt was from the encourage-ment Michael and Lily gave me. After twelve hours of intense labor, our little five-and-a-half-pound Aurianna Miranda was born.

It was only the beginning of a horrible hospital stay. Because we weren't assertive enough, the hospital staff seemed to take advan-tage of us. Babies' temperature regulating mechanisms don't work well the first twenty-four hours, so the nurses put a lot of blankets on Aurianna. Her temperature increased. Because they were con-cerned about infection, they immediately did bladder and spinal taps, administered antibiotics and told me there was a chance Aurianna had spinal meningitis. When we asked the doctor about the test results, he said that all the tests were negative and that there had just been too many blankets on her.

Giving up our plans for a homebirth, combined with a traumatic hospital experience, was one of the biggest shocks of our lives. We decided that if we ever had another baby, things would be a lot different.

❧          ❧          ❧

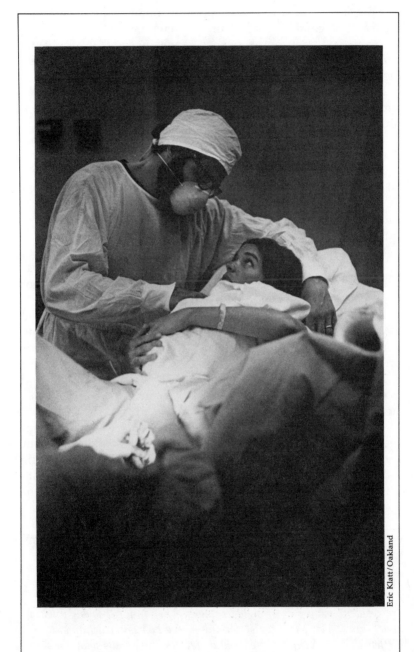

Wow, pregnant again! We began planning a homebirth immediately. A good diet and plenty of exercise were the main goals. We arranged for my mother to spend some time with us before and after the due date of October 7. We chose the birth team. We could then relax and enjoy the pregnancy while our baby grew.

By September the Braxton-Hicks contractions were getting strong. I felt twinges in my cervix. An examination revealed thinning out, so it could be any time.

October came and still no baby. We were going to make the due date after all.

It was October 10 and we wanted our baby out! We decided to take a ride to the ocean. We spent time walking and had a delicious dinner before our return home. Perhaps it was the change in elevation from sea level to the ridge top, but at the summit my water broke.

We arrived home at 8:00 p.m. and contacted Lily and my friend, Kathy, to inform them that this could be the night. My mother was already with us. Michael and I took a walk and prayed that labor would begin soon.

At 11:00 p.m. I began to feel the first real contractions. We tried to get some sleep, but by 3:00 a.m. the contractions were getting stronger. At 7:00 a.m. we decided it was time to round everyone up.

Lily arrived at 9:30. She did a cervical examination and found that I was 6-7 centimeters dilated. Kathy came at 10:00 and an hour later Rebecca, my other midwife, showed up. By then I was 10 centimeters dilated and felt like pushing. This was when I appreciated the entire birth team most of all. It took almost an hour and a half of pushing. Being exhausted, I depended on everyone to help maneuver and hold me in the many positions needed to bring the baby out. At 12:32 p.m. our wonderful Micah David greeted us.

I never thought I'd say childbirth was fun, but with the support of Michael, two-year-old Aurianna, Lily, Kathy, Rebecca, my mother, and most important Jehovah God, Micah's birth was a real pleasure.

*Mary resides with her husband and children in a small town where they are resident managers of eight cottages. The family enjoys gardening and fishing. Mary is a registered nurse and has assisted Lily at homebirths, coached friends at hospital deliveries and enjoys photographing births.*

# The Tale of Buddy and Rose

by Karen Rosen

August first, the due date, came and went. How much longer—a day, a week, a month? My sister-in-law Jody and my husband Mark were more excited than I, watching my every move to the point that any "ooh" or "ahh" I uttered was taken as a sign of impending labor. On Monday, the sixth, Jody and I went to town. On our way home the lower back cramps I'd been experiencing all morning turned into regular light contractions. So this was it. I'd read and heard a lot about what could happen, yet it was all such a mystery. Would it hurt? Would I be able to integrate the feelings to the level beyond pain as other women had?

The contractions continued all afternoon. By 6:30 p.m. they were five to seven minutes apart and quite regular, so we called the midwives. At 8:00 Kate and Kathleen arrived and suggested that I try to sleep to store up energy for when I would need it—they would spend the night. Maybe I should have started concentrating on the contractions from the start and not spent the night trying to keep everything low-key.

At 2:00 a.m. I woke Kathleen up to be with me during the contractions as they were getting harder to handle on my own. I was able to doze for the five minutes between contractions and would wake up during each one for deep chest breathing.

By morning I was not much further along: 4-5 centimeters dilated, so Kate went to the Clinic for her morning appointments. When she returned at noon, my dilation hadn't increased. We decided she should break my water bag, hoping that would cause me to dilate further. It only helped a little, and by then I was getting quite tired.

The afternoon progressed faster than I did. I was getting so tired, and things were moving along so slowly, that the thought of a cesarean section crossed my mind. By that evening, talk of going to the hospital began in earnest. Could I think of any reasons that were keeping me from dilating? I was getting a little scared and could feel the tension in my cervix as each contraction came and went. It definitely wasn't opening up no matter how I tried to relax. We decided to go to the hospital, hoping a muscle relaxant would help me open the rest of the way. I felt apprehensive at first until I heard that Dr. Bill would be there.

The full moon was rising as we started toward town. Bouncing in the back of the station wagon brought on the urge to push. Kathleen thought that possibly I had finished dilating. However, by the time we made it through the maze of police cars and emergency vehicles which were unusually plentiful at the hospital that night, Dr. Bill found that my 7-centimeter dilation had closed back down to 5 centimeters, and my cervix was getting swollen.

After what seemed like a long time, I finally got a muscle relaxant, and I spent an hour blowing and relaxing only to find my cervix still in the same condition. The decision to do a cesarean was made.

With no anesthesiologist at the local hospital, I would have to go to a larger hospital an hour away. I couldn't believe we'd have to drive there as it seemed that I couldn't keep on blowing much longer—I wanted the c-section done right away! Expecting a streamline ambulance ride, I decided against leaving right away in our station wagon. If only I'd known—it ended up taking two hours to get me into the ambulance and on our way.

Eighty miles an hour, bumps, stops to take my blood pressure, hitting a ditch and being thrown off the stretcher—time seemed unreal. I knew I had to keep blowing, but I didn't know where my strength would come from. Kathleen was invaluable, keeping me in touch with reality. The urge to bear down was so strong, yet the fear of tearing my cervix and pushing on the baby helped me to keep blowing.

We arrived at the hospital around 2:00 a.m. After a quick check by the doctor, the nurses started to prepare me for surgery. Luckily the doctor knew it was not necessary to x-ray or fool around trying to figure out why I wasn't dilating.

Things now took on the quality of a television show with me as the main character. Actually, things usually go smoother on television. One nurse was *trying* to put in an IV while another was *trying* to shave my abdomen. Yet another nurse was *trying* to insert a catheter between contractions, which at that point were half a minute apart and would sometimes just run together. There were two different people asking me the same questions at different times. It was crazy!

At last they were ready for me in surgery. They would only let

Mark and Kathleen come with me as far as the doors of the operating room, and from there I was blowing on my own until I could catch the hand of one of the nurses as she whisked by—I had to hold on tight not to lose her. Monitors were taped all over my body, I was hooked up to machines—it was scary as I had not even considered the possibility of going to the hospital or of having a cesarean. It was comforting to know that the baby's heart was beating strongly. They set up a tent between my head and my belly and put an oxygen mask on me. It was hard to blow with it on, and I had to push it away once or twice to catch a breath. Finally, I was put to sleep—my labor was over!

They pulled the baby out with forceps at 2:52 a.m. I came to in the recovery room at 4:10. Mark told me our son was fine. His head was slightly elongated, and his eyes were puffed shut from being pushed against my cervix for so long. He also had two marks on his cheeks from the forceps. I saw none of this as they wheeled me by the nursery on the way to my bed. The nurses brought him to me at 6:30 a.m. and he looked fine by then. I was so worn out from the past forty hours that I didn't mind not having the baby with me.

The pain I felt from the surgery and from my uterus contracting made the labor seem like the easier part, although the pain killers they gave me worked wonders. It was hard to make those first few trips to the bathroom after the catheter was removed. It felt like the incision across my belly was going to split open. Finding a comfortable way to nurse was a feat, and switching the baby from one breast to the other was even harder.

But time heals all wounds and mine healed fast. It took about two weeks until I could really move around or carry the baby. It took about six months for us to decide on a name for him and nine until I was pregnant again. We wanted to have two children close together, so . . .

🐦       🐦       🐦

I had heard so much about women attempting a vaginal birth after a cesarean that I decided to give it a try. Mark was away with Buddy, our son, giving me a break two weeks before my due date. Much to my dismay, I woke up one morning at 2:00 with strange cramps in my lower back. As I gained consciousness, I realized they were coming in waves, every ten minutes. I had no way to reach Mark until later that morning, and since he was three thousand miles away, I knew it would have to be a very long labor or he would miss it.

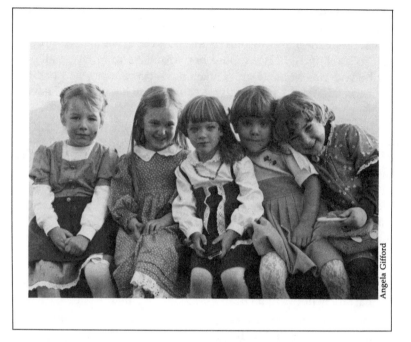

Angela Gifford

Luckily, Mark's sister and her friend were staying with me. One of them went to get my midwife, Kathleen, and then we all drove to the town where the hospital is located. We checked into a motel for the early part of my labor, not wanting to get hooked up to the monitors too early. Everything went along smoothly—nice regular easy contractions. We went to the hospital in the early afternoon, and I got settled and hooked up to a fetal heart monitor.

By 6:00 p.m. I had reached 7 centimeters. When 7:00 arrived and I was still at 7 centimeters and had the urge to push, I started to feel defeated. The doctor came in, and we both felt I had been trying long enough, so we decided to do another cesarean.

This time I had a spinal anesthetic instead of a general. Kathleen was allowed into surgery with me since Mark wasn't there, and she had taken the required class for anyone attending a c-section. She stood by my head as the doctor pushed my baby girl out. Kathleen held her next to me so I could wrap my free arm around her. The baby was so beautiful, dark and hairy. The pushing that the doctor did, described as pressure by some women, was somewhat painful, as was getting stitched up afterwards. I was so thankful I was awake to see and touch Rose when she was born, because she came down with pneumonia hours after her birth, and they had to shave her head to put in an IV. But that's another story.

While some people don't want anything to do with modern technology when it comes to birthing their babies, I'm thankful it's available as I wouldn't be here to tell the tale without it. I now have two healthy children to spend my time with.

*Karen lives with her husband and two children and has part-time care of three stepchildren. She spends her free time gardening, working in their small vineyard and raising goats and angora rabbits. She helped establish an art center where she works in the pottery studio.*

# A Letter

by Barbara Anthony

---

Dear Chaya Rose:

You were born at 3:42 on the afternoon of September 15th. What a year to remember. It started in Los Angeles. There I was, New Year's Eve with your dad. Don't know how we got together because we hadn't seen each other in a long time. Must have been to make you! Happy New Year.

Nine months you rode inside. Up and down, as you well know, on the roller coaster of emotions. Thank God we were protected from the abortion that came so close.

Moved back to the hills of Northern California at seven months for the love and support of old friends. Lots of sun and swimming through the embryonic fluid of forever until the eve of your birth. A stomach full of baby and exotic hors d'oeuvres woke me at 3:00 a.m. with strangely rhythmic gas pains.

I phoned Kate, our midwife, and started panicking after the tenth ring. *Hello?* "Hello, this is Barbara." *Who?* Oh, God, she doesn't remember me . . . "Something's happening—feelings," (not wanting to call them contractions). *OK, I'll be up in a while.*

She arrived and examined me. 1 centimeter. "What does that mean?" *You're in early labor.* Oh, no! Am I ready for this?

Kathy, my breathing coach, arrived along with another friend. Couldn't handle the energy of an additional person, so we asked her to leave. Felt like I had to laugh and entertain when I really felt like falling apart. Cried long and hard in my midwife's arms. Dear friend, I am afraid. The contractions were getting stronger and closer together. Time now to work with Kathy, learning to breathe together. Actually, I wasn't really breathing like they taught us in class. I went in for moaning and gasping. Spent a good deal of time in the bathtub. The hot water felt good, and the contractions seemed easier. About six hours into the labor, my mucus plug came out. Amazing substance.

In the living room, Kathy suggested I play the piano. I'd get into some dramatic movement and then stop for an equally dramatic contraction. I'm a Leo.

It was intense. Not pain, but the pressure of things pushing and

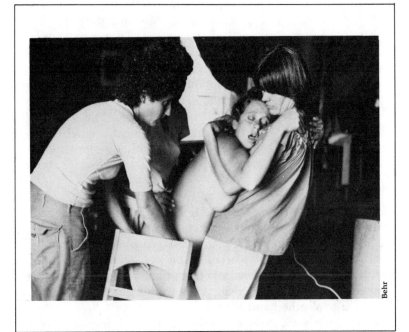

Behr

stretching parts of me that had never been stretched. Crying out,
touch these places—HARD—contractions back to back now. On
hands and knees, trying to run away, with no place to go except
through it; and suddenly I felt like pushing. Pushing already? I was
examined and my cervix was almost completely dilated. Get ready!

We were on the first floor and our lovely room, all set and
waiting for you, was on the third floor. Make up your mind *now!*
So I took a deep breath and raced up the stairs to the mezzanine,
dropped to my knees for a contraction, and then on to the third
floor for the most incredible experience of my life—you.

Unaware that all of our friends had arrived, I focused my total
self on pushing. Working together, you and I, pushing you through
the tunnel to your new life. Push, push. *Good, you're doing good,*
someone said. *Reach down. Feel your baby coming.*

The sac that held you hadn't broken yet, and I could feel it. Oh,
I can't believe it! Push again. Touch. Feel how close. Purple face.
Push, push. Roar. I feel you coming. Look, there's the bubble.
There was meconium in the water so we popped the bubble. Pssst.
Water everywhere. Less pressure. Push again. How many more?
*Maybe ten more.* Oh, no. So I pushed with all of my strength. Three

more contractions and you were crowning. *OK, stop pushing now — just blow.* Burning. Oh, it hurts. My eyes were tightly shut then. *Barbara! Open your eyes and look at your baby.* There was your little head sticking out from between my legs. While I watched, wide-eyed and unbelieving, you extended a hand to pull yourself out. Then your body spiralled, swam out, and there you were, staring at me. Face to face after such a long time.

"Hello, I'm Barbara and I'm your mother." I told you of the wonders of this life; of your strength and what a good time we were going to have. You looked up at me with pure love and faith shining in your eyes. You're so beautiful. Tender loving wonder. Welcome.

Turned out you were a girl and I was glad. Held you for a long time and then I cut the cord. The first step on our separate paths. I miss you already. You wouldn't suckle at my breast to bring on the final contractions for the placenta. So Auntie Fox did, and you went to take a bath. The placenta came out, whole and healthy. I hadn't torn at all (you were only five pounds — thanks for making it so easy on me). I felt great. After twelve hours of exhausting work, I felt refreshed and alive.

Took a long hot shower and afterwards was sitting on the couch awaiting your return from the bath — and you came, with a little peep of recognition. Holding you at my breast, the joy over-whelmed me and I cried.

My beautiful daughter.

That was one year ago, and we've laughed and cried many times together. I just want you to know that I'm with you, and if sometimes you don't think I am, it just might be that I don't know what to say or what to do. I am growing up with you, too. And I promise you, Chaya Rose, that I shall always listen as best I can, and help you with all of my heart. I love you today and for always.

Mom

*Barbara and Chaya now live in the country near Santa Fe, New Mexico. Barbara reports that Chaya, who helps gather firewood, cleans her own room and empties the compost, has changed from a baby into a little girl. She writes, "I remember a dream I had when I was pregnant. The baby was already born and nursing at my breast. I was surprised that she already had teeth and as I looked down, she began to grow and grow until her feet touched the ground. She got up and walked out of the room, away from me, as I called, 'But you're too young . . . ' Now I understand how my mother can still say, 'Somehow, you'll always be my baby.'"*

# Rainbow Warrior

## by Agnes Cereceda

Even though it was my third pregnancy, I was a little apprehensive as my other children were nine and twelve years old. My first child was born under barbaric conditions in Los Angeles. Fourteen hours after the birth I begged to see my baby, whom the nurses finally brought to me. He and I were both new to nursing (not one of the other twenty-five women who had just had their babies was breastfeeding), so when he didn't nurse right away, they immediately took him back to the nursery. I cried and begged for my baby—they brought me tranquilizers. They thought that I was a "bad" mother because I wanted to nurse my baby and refused to have him circumcised. I wanted to go home but Zachary became jaundiced and had to have a blood transfusion. How can anyone bond under those conditions?

I was only twenty years old, but my instincts guided me. I went home without my baby, but for the next four days while he was in the hospital, and I was not allowed to nurse him, I pumped my milk every two hours with a store-bought hand pump. When he could finally leave the hospital, I refused to take bottles home with me, and I nursed him until he was a year old. Despite my efforts, we were never really bonded, and he now lives with his father.

Several years after Zachary's birth I found myself pregnant again, and I knew there had to be a better way of birthing. We had moved from Los Angeles, and I found only one doctor in our community who would allow natural childbirth and permit fathers in the delivery room. Even though it was a hospital birth, the experience was very high, and I felt so good afterwards. We bonded very strongly, and I nursed my daughter, Sunshine, until she was two and a half years old.

Nine years later, after settling down in Northern California with my daughter and a new man, Lon, we discovered I was pregnant while we were still discovering ourselves. I was happy to be having a baby. I firmly believe that the spirit of your child is with you from the time of conception, and if you are happy and full of love, your baby will be too. I was concerned for Lon, though. I wasn't sure how he would handle the pregnancy.

I had never been to the Clinic before but went in one Wednesday (prenatal day) and complained that I had gained three pounds. Alison, who was taking my blood pressure, said, "Honey, I gained seventy pounds with my kids." I was amazed by this beautiful lady, full of light and love—the most clear-eyed person I'd seen in a while. I next met Lorraine and Becca. They spent forty-five minutes with me, listening to my complaints, wiping away my tears, and reassuring me that my anxieties, fears and hopes were not going to harm my baby but were normal and that it was OK to have such feelings.

With this pregnancy I felt tired a lot, but whenever I saw one of the midwives—it didn't matter which one—she would zap me with some energy. One day I was feeling lousy with a toothache and was going through emotional upheavals. When I walked into the Clinic, every midwife hugged me and gave me so much energy that three days later I was still feeling it.

I grew so big that many people thought I was going to have twins. "No," I would say, "just one big baby." The due date was on a Wednesday, so I made the twenty-five mile trip to town for my prenatal appointment. I didn't feel like going because we had to travel five miles on a bumpy dirt road, and toward the end of my pregnancy every time I drove over it I would have crazy contractions that I knew didn't mean anything. When we were almost to town, I wanted to turn around and go home. I wasn't in labor—I just wanted to be home. I went on anyway and kept my appointment with Dr. Bill.

I had asked Lorraine to be at the birth. When I saw her in the back of the Clinic that day, I just waved. She told me later that when I didn't go back and talk with her but waved and left, I looked like a lady who just wanted to go home and have her baby. She knew I would be having my baby that night.

We went to eat at a restaurant, and I was feeling uncomfortable. I was so big I couldn't fit into the booth. I started having those crazy contractions again. The waitress came up and asked, "When's that baby due?"

"Today, right now!" I responded. She must have thought I meant that it was coming right then, because her eyes grew bigger than her glasses, and her hand touched her mouth with a big "Oh!"

My urge to go home became very strong. Once there, I settled down and started quilting a baby blanket. I kept quilting, breathing faster and slower and not paying any attention. Lon came in, heard my breathing and asked, "Are you having the baby or what?"

"Oh, no," I told him.

"Why are you breathing that way?" he asked.

"What way?" I wondered. It was then I realized I was having contractions and they were two minutes apart. I finally started to believe what I had been telling people all day: I was having my baby!

It was after 10:00 p.m., and Lon had to call on the CB radio to a neighbor who could relay a message to Lorraine and Becca. The contractions were strong and intense, especially in my lower back. I wished I hadn't been so foolish and waited so long, because I knew it would be at least an hour before the midwives would come.

Becca and Lorraine arrived at 11:45 p.m. After setting things up, Lorraine checked me, and I was almost fully dilated, ready for transition. Oh boy, I thought, almost done. My transition had only been nine minutes with Sunshine, who was now on the stairs that overlooked our bed. I was so happy to be at home having my baby. I felt higher than I could ever remember. But I knew I had a lot of hard work still ahead of me.

The baby was having a difficult time coming down the birth canal. Lorraine and Becca had me get up on my knees and hang on to Lon. Around 2:00 a.m. they had me sit up, and it felt so good. When I was on my knees, the pain in my lower back was very intense. Becca massaged and pressed down on my back to relieve the pain. She worked hard, and it really shows in the pictures a friend took.

Once I was sitting up, I wanted to push, but I could feel that the baby's head was really big. I knew it would take more than a couple of good shoves to get it out. I pushed, and I pushed, and I pushed with Lorraine breathing and blowing with me, looking me in the eye, guiding me, giving me her strength and trust. "Push, Agnes, push, push!" chanted Becca. I howled and howled and then—*Pop!*—the head came out into Lon's hands. Becca removed the cord from around the baby's neck, and I gave one more big shove, and the biggest thing ever to come through me came out! They put him on my belly, and he immediately squirmed to my breast and started nursing. "Well, here I am, Mom!" I started to pat him slowly. He felt huge: ten pounds, four ounces; twenty-two inches long. I had only one little tear. I was so happy.

After the cord was cut, Lon and Sunshine took him outside where the full moon was shining. I started to cry, I felt so lucky. I

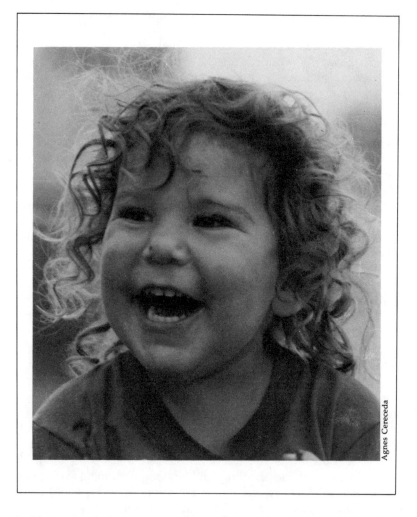

Agnes Cereceda

held my new baby, knowing that God must really love me. Marley was born at 2:21 a.m. and by 3:30 the midwives were gone, and he was asleep between Lon and me in bed. It felt very special.

I had been in labor for six hours, and most of it was heavy and intense. I couldn't have done it so well without Lon. One of the things I've learned is not to underestimate the strength and power of the "be-here-now" attitude in the father of your baby. The birthing experience is very "here" and "now." To open and share it with the people you love brings you the strength and energy to carry through. No matter what happened in the past or what might lie ahead in the future, the shared birth experience creates a bond.

Marley is now seventeen months old and very big. We sit and watch him waddle his way around the house, curls bopping on his head, full of smiles and laughter. The sparkle in his eyes shows his love, and as we look at him, we see the love we have—for him, for each other, our children and family, for all living creatures, Mother Earth, the universe, and the Great Spirit.

*Agnes, who originates from Ecuador, lives with two of her children as close to nature as possible. She is an environmental activist and has spent the past five years trying to save a wilderness area from destruction. She says, "It is important that our children experience Mother Earth the way God created it, not the way man has destroyed it." She also works closely with Native American issues and indigenous people's struggles. In her spare time Agnes is a shoemaker, beadwork artist and an award-winning photographer.*

# Two Different Births

by Mary Neufeld

My first pregnancy was quite a surprise from the beginning to the end. I didn't realize that I was pregnant until I was two and a half months along. I had a regular period the first month and a lighter one the second month. When my "tummy aches" weren't relieved after a week of milk of magnesia, my husband Harold and I finally realized I was pregnant. I was quite surprised, then felt myself getting into the spirit of what millions of women over the ages have experienced.

My doctor was also surprised that I was able to get pregnant because of my past history of severe pelvic inflammatory disease as a result of using an IUD. We were worried about my pregnancy and wondered if its continuation would have a negative effect on my health, but our fears were unfounded.

My pregnancy progressed very well. The birthing day, however, came unexpectedly soon. Though I was tired, I had a workaholic drive to get the house we were building as complete as possible. I was doing carpentry work and was cramped in a small space for a few hours. My water started to leak so I stopped working. I didn't feel any contractions, though, so I didn't know what it meant. It was the beginning of August and the baby wasn't due until the end of September. Later that night my water broke completely, and I began having contractions five minutes apart. We couldn't believe my labor was starting.

We got to the hospital at 3:30 a.m. We were supposed to start taking the Lamaze and prenatal classes that day, so we had to learn the breathing on the spot. The breathing exercises helped to keep me calm. Harold was a great coach, and I was most comfortable being alone with him.

It was all so exciting—even though I knew that the baby was six weeks premature, I felt it was going to be a healthy baby. It was a busy night for the obstetric ward as six other babies were born. After the last baby was delivered, the doctor came in to check my cervix and was surprised to find I was fully dilated. My transition had been smooth, like the waves of an ocean with which I had flowed.

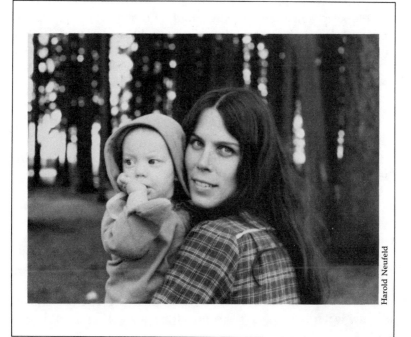

Harold Neufeld

I was wheeled to the delivery room at 9:30 a.m. I had to ask the doctors and nurses to remove their surgical masks because I have a hearing impairment and need to lip-read. Harold went to put his surgical gown on, and as soon as he came back I started to push. The doctor said he had to give me a small episiotomy for the baby's sake. After two more pushes Carl was out and crying. The umbilical cord was fascinating—it was so big and perfectly spiral. The doctor cut it immediately, and the nurses put Carl in an incubator.

My expectations were shattered. I had planned on having the baby in the labor room and keeping him with me after the birth. I hadn't planned on having an episiotomy nor on having the umbilical cord cut before it stopped pulsing. Everything that happened was beyond my control because he was premature. He weighed over five pounds so he didn't have to stay in the hospital for long. Within twelve hours of his birth he was no longer receiving oxygen, and the IV and the heart monitor were taken off.

On the third day he became jaundiced and needed Bilirubin lights. I had some difficulty in nursing as he was so small and weak, and my nipples seemed so big. I was up all night trying to nurse him every hour because he wasn't getting enough nourishment to keep him asleep for any length of time. The next morning I was frazzled, but a nurse who saw my problem gave Carl a bottle of water, which worked really well.

Although Carl's birth didn't meet my expectations, I was happy and relieved to be taking home a healthy baby. Harold, Carl and I were now a family.

❦    ❦    ❦

My second pregnancy was quite different. It was planned, and since I knew what symptoms to look for, I knew I was pregnant by the time I was one and a half months along. Compared to my first pregnancy, which my friends like to tease me about lasting only four and a half months, this pregnancy seemed very long. I was two weeks overdue—I was so much bigger than before and very uncomfortable.

One morning I decided to take two tablespoons of castor oil, hoping it would start my labor. Harold was installing a CB in the car, and I went outside to hurry him along. Just as he finished, I started having contractions five minutes apart. Forty-five minutes later my water broke, and the contractions took on a greater intensity.

We got in the car and headed toward the hospital. The drive on the dirt road was uncomfortable, and I asked Harold to stop during contractions. It was funny watching him try to coach and drive at the same time. The contractions were getting so close together we called on the CB for an ambulance and my midwife. I was afraid we wouldn't make it to the hospital in time. I was in transition and falling asleep between contractions.

By coincidence we met the ambulance and my midwife, Mary, at the same time. Mary and I got into the ambulance, and Harold followed in the car. (Later I wished he had come with us.) When Mary checked me, I was fully dilated. I wanted to start pushing, but Mary suggested that I wait until we got to the hospital where it would be more comfortable and Harold would be there. Mary was so helpful in coaching the pant-blow breathing—if I hadn't met her and the ambulance, I probably would have had the baby in the car.

When we arrived at the hospital, Dr. Bill was there, and the birthing room was ready. I felt hot, took my clothes off, jumped on the bed and started pushing. With the fifth push Loren was born. We were able to wait for the umbilical cord to stop pulsing, and Harold cut it. I held the baby and bonded with him. He started nursing right away and kept it up for a few hours before he fell asleep for the night.

It was a much more "normal" birth than my first, although the ride was pretty hectic. My labor lasted three hours—it was so easy we could have stayed home, but that's using hindsight.

On the way home the next day we saw a newborn baby deer, still wet from his birth, wobble into a ditch, curl up, and watch us drive by. It was beautiful and seemed quite appropriate for Loren's homecoming.

*Mary grew up in the suburbs of Detroit. She left college and moved to California when an administrator discouraged her from pursuing her career goals because of her hearing disability. She was impressed with the self-sufficient lifestyle of friends she visited in the country and decided to buy land and build her own home. Since marrying Harold, Mary spends her time raising their children, tending the animals and garden and growing unusual varieties of irises.*

# A Reason for Pain: Anders and Leif

by Kathy Holtermann

---

I had a normal pregnancy. By the end I was uncomfortable and emotionally ready to give birth. I wanted my body to get back to its normal state. I had gained forty pounds, had heartburn and could never find a comfortable position—standing, sitting or lying down.

My labor started one morning at 6:30. I knew that something was going to happen and I should go to the toilet. I had a strange feeling, as if a bubble was growing in my vagina. It grew and grew until it popped with a small bang. Then I had strong cramps and contractions. I called my sister and timed the contractions. By 7:00 a.m. they were seconds apart, and my husband Jay called the midwives.

I well remember giving birth because it was an overwhelming experience—it was terribly painful. I continued to have cramps and contractions, and my pubic bone ached as if it was expanding and opening up while the baby moved downward. Every time I moved I had a strong contraction and I had to freeze and sit down. I spent most of the first four hours sitting on the toilet. Each time I got up, I would have another contraction. Sometimes I walked into the next room where everyone was eating breakfast. They all stopped eating and watched me expectantly as I ran back into the bathroom. One of the three midwives and one of my sisters would come into the bathroom to see if everything was OK.

When I was 6 centimeters dilated I went to lie down on the bed. The need to push came soon and it was overwhelming. I had to use all my willpower and concentration not to push. It felt as if the baby was doing the pushing, and I had to fight it. It was very painful. I was so grateful when I was 10 centimeters dilated and I could push.

One thought that occurred to me was that I was going to die. I was so tired of the pain. I remembered something that my mother had told me when I was a little girl. She said, "Never be afraid of pain. Accept it and try to understand it. It is there for a reason. If

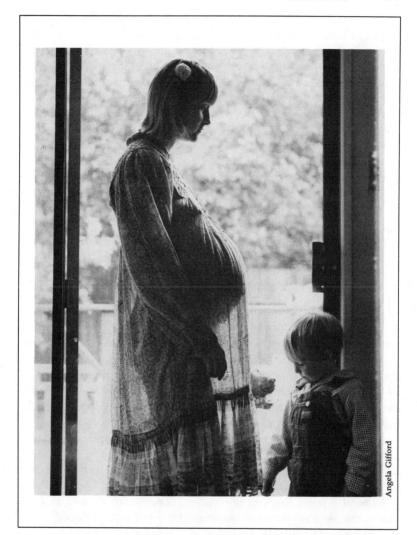

Angela Gifford

the pain is too great to bear, then God will put you to sleep and you will die and have no more pain." Well, I didn't want to die but to give birth. I let go of the fear. In the next few minutes my son's head popped out and I was so happy. The midwives suctioned his nose and mouth. Jay was there to catch him as he came out. It was 12:30 p.m., December 20. He was beautiful and he looked up at me as if to say, *I know you and I'm glad to see you.*

My son's head and body had come out very fast. The top of his head came first instead of the crown, and both shoulders came out at once instead of one at a time. I had a third degree tear, from the top of my urethra to my anus, and I was bleeding heavily. After I held and nursed my baby, I was rushed to a hospital where the doctor spent an hour stitching me.

When we returned to our home, it had been cleaned up, and my bed was waiting for me. My son was crying, but we were all happy. For a few days I could not sit up or walk standing straight. It hurt just to move, and stung to pee. I took hot sitz baths with comfrey leaves every other hour to aid the healing. I wasn't able to take care of myself or my baby. My husband, my mother and my three sisters shared the task of caring for us. I was so grateful that I could nurse Anders. It was our first Christmas together as a family and a wonderful time for me.

ॐ     ॐ     ॐ

Three years later after moving to the country, I found myself pregnant again. This pregnancy progressed normally and I was happy to be having a second child.

One midnight, I awoke with a strange feeling of pulsing in my cervix, an opening up. It was strong and definite—I knew I was dilating and that this was labor. I called Lorraine, my midwife, and she told me to take a warm bath to slow the labor down. Since I'd had a six-hour labor with my first birth, she thought that this labor would be very short, and we were worried that the baby might come before she arrived.

My mother, my twin sister Mimi, and her one-and-a-half-year-old daughter, Mia, had come to be with me for the birth. I called my husband and the friends who were to attend the birth, and they arrived along with Lorraine as I relaxed in the tub.

When Lorraine checked me, I was 8 centimeters dilated and felt like vomiting. Everyone circled around me as I sat on my bed doing the "panting" breath. Being watched while I was in pain made me feel uncomfortable, but I was too busy to think much about it. Suddenly I felt that something was going to happen and I ran to the toilet—my water broke. I spent the next hour dashing between the bed and the toilet. Little Mia followed me with wonder, confusion and concern. Seeing Lorraine wipe the sweat from my face, she tried to imitate her. With a warm washcloth she would gently wipe my knee, then look up to see if she had comforted me; this gave me joy.

My friend Karen sat close to me and helped me to stay focused on my breathing. Push! Push! Ow, it hurts! Push! I wondered, When will this end? I knelt on the floor with my head resting on the bed as I pushed. Soon I gave birth to my second son. It was 2:27 a.m.; the labor had taken less than three hours.

We had talked to our three-year-old son Anders in detail about the impending birth. We bought books, drew pictures and explained it to him. He was asleep during most of my labor, and I was glad. I asked that he be woken when the baby's head crowned. He came into the room tired and was very worried about me when he saw all the blood. After I gave birth, he was concerned about the umbilical cord coming from my vagina, but he didn't cry. Soon we were all lying in bed admiring our new baby as I nursed him.

I tore again, although not as badly as with my first birth. It was snowing as I was taken to the Clinic to be stitched; I hated to leave my baby. Three hours later when I came home, I noticed just how special my new baby, Leif, was. His soul had not made the transition to earth yet; part of him was still in heaven. I felt blessed during the next week as I watched him come into his body.

*Kathy, now a single parent, originates from Sweden. She graduated from the University of California at Berkeley with a degree in Scandinavian Studies. Her interests include beading, needlework and gardening, and when her children are older she hopes to resume jogging, marathon running and backpacking.*

# The Unexpected

by Judi Horvath

I had finally started labor, two weeks past the due date. What a wonderful pregnancy it had been—so smooth, so easy. I'd had polyhydromnios, but the results of a sonogram reassured us that the baby was fine, and the condition cleared up by the due date.

My friends were gathered nearby along with my husband Charlie and our midwife. All had been hovering close for so long. I had so much support and love. Because we live an hour and a half from the hospital, we were spending the early part of the labor at a motel that was only five minutes away. We felt so secure, so covered.

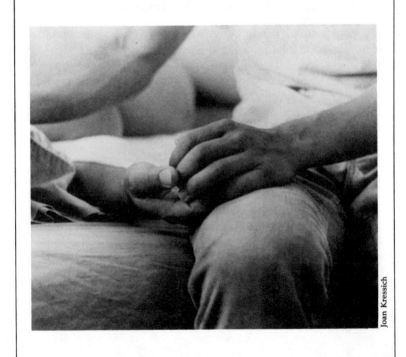

Joan Kressich

Labor was progressing nicely. I had back labor, the baby being posterior. We listened for the baby's heartbeat and heard it. I got up to go to the bathroom, and while I was sitting on the toilet I felt our baby tumble around inside me. Another contraction came and went. We listened for the heartbeat again—none, we couldn't hear it.

Charlie loaded the car in a matter of minutes, and we were off to the hospital. They listened for a heartbeat—none. I was 8 centimeters dilated. They put me on the delivery table, did an episiotomy and with forceps pulled Benjamin from me. I got a glimpse of him as he was handed to the pediatrician. He was covered with dark green meconium. Charlie and I had our heads together as they worked to revive him. It had been so long since he had received oxygen. Later the autopsy report said, "Cause of Death: Occult umbilical prolapse."

Numbness. Someone else's movie. We saw Benjamin's peaceful face, touched him, and then he was gone. Such a deep, profound emptiness I had never known. Charlie and I were alone in the hospital room trying to find a way to communicate. It finally came while we shared some food. Then we had to phone our parents to tell them that our baby Benjamin had died. From there on it became a reality that we have both had to deal with.

It's been quite a roller coaster ride, highs and lows, a ride I'm sure I'll be on for the rest of my life. I feel very lucky that we've been able to talk to each other—to say all the things that needed to be said out loud. I find that if I don't talk about it to someone now and then and see their face react and hear them respond to me, I begin to think I made the whole thing up. How could it have happened to us?

We've learned so much, and after two years I continue to learn. Benjamin was an individual with choices and decisions to make. I have only so much control; some things I have to accept. As hard as it was for me to let go, I will always have those nine close months to remember and cherish. We often think of him as a higher being who only had to spend nine months here. We will always miss him and love him.

*Two and a half years later, after a miscarriage, Judi delivered a healthy baby girl by cesarean section. She now teaches first grade at a community school and is working toward certification in Montessori education. She says, "I love exercising and dancing, but mostly I am in awe and feel blessed that our daughter Bree Anna has come to be with Charlie and me."*

how hard it is to understand
why birth and death are one

yet he knew
what he had to know
and we accept, with tears,
the lesson of this turning

so, has he not taught us,
and has he not brought us
another step
   to our own passage
      into the fields of light
         and higher pastures of love

We thank you little Pisces boy.


                    From a friend,
                    Rod Algoet

# Birth Dance

## by Susan Alban Stoft

I must begin by saying I have a very strange body. With a thirty-two-inch hip measurement and a bent posture, I had always imagined that I would have to have my children by cesarean. But at the age of twenty-eight, as the birth of my first child drew closer, I knew I didn't want a hospital experience.

The pregnancy progressed fine and I felt great. Then, six weeks before the due date, my little person inside decided to become breech. Until then my husband Wesley and I had planned a home-birth with a midwife. Suddenly, everything changed. Each doctor we saw, after taking one look at my unusual body, said he'd gladly schedule me for a c-section any time I liked. Luckily, after a long search, we found a doctor who agreed to let me attempt a vaginal birth provided all his criteria were met: I could not be anemic; it could not be a footling breech; it would have to be a natural unmedicated birth because he wanted me to be aware of what was happening so I could help him deliver the baby. I felt I could accept his conditions.

A week before I was due, I went into labor following a slow and warm lovemaking with Wesley. *Oh no, I'm not ready for this!* was my first reaction. But, indeed it was amniotic waters leaking out. The doctor wanted me to come to the hospital right away so he could check to make sure that the baby wasn't a footling breech. They x-rayed me to see if the head would fit through my pelvis, and lo and behold, there was a nice wide opening within my tiny hips. The doctor said that we'd give it a try, but if the baby was not born within twenty-four hours, I would have to have a cesarean. I accepted this with quiet patience. We walked up and down the halls of the hospital so the weight of the baby would help to dilate my cervix. I stopped with each contraction to breathe deeply. I was amazed by the flush of heat that came after each wave, showing me that my body was working hard and doing what it knew how to do.

All day long we walked the halls, longing to be outside in the fresh air. Finally I went back to the newly set up birthing room and hung up my familiar god's eyes and Tibetan marriage thanka.

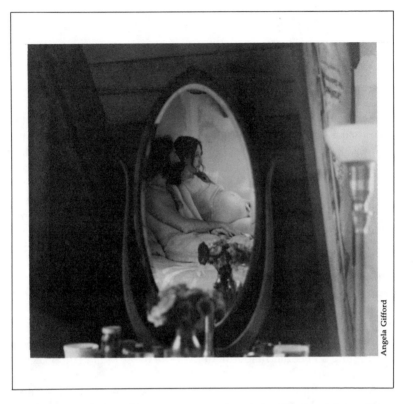

Angela Gifford

Wesley climbed into bed with me and together we experienced my labor. I thought, It's not too bad—it's very interesting to watch my body do this incredible birth dance to let my little one out.

The night wore on, and an old friend and our birth class instructor came in to assist me. The nurse insisted on putting a fetal heart monitor around my belly. Watching the peaks of my contractions was interesting for a while, but since it was the wee hours of the night and everyone was tired, I suggested that they lie on the floor and sleep; I wanted to be alone.

I lay on my side and dozed between contractions. The last time the nurse checked me, I was 7 centimeters. As I watched the monitor, I saw it register double peaks of contractions. They were very powerful but exhilarating. I must have been in this state for hours: dozing in dreamland to rise steadily into reality with each contraction, only to slip back into total relaxation. I kept waiting for the legendary transition, expecting it to be psychedelic, but instead it just slowly turned into pushing. I wasn't consciously pushing; I was observing my uterus push. This went on for some time until suddenly I felt pressure on the base of my spine.

"Uh, wake up! I think the nurse should check me," I said. Everyone jumped up and someone rushed out. The nurse came in, took one look at me and ran out saying, "Oh my, the baby is coming!" There was immediate panic. No one was ready and the doctor wasn't even there. They wheeled me to the delivery room and made Wesley put on a surgical gown and mask. His beard stuck out of the mask and flowed down his gown. The doctor on duty stood in the corner with his arms crossed, looking at me as if he was thinking, *Don't do this to me, lady.* I had to lie on the table with my knees pressed together and pant every time a contraction came because no one wanted to deal with my little breech baby. Luckily, my doctor lived nearby and since it was 5:00 a.m., he was able to streak through town. It seemed like a long time to me, but my friends were there to remind me to pant.

When the doctor arrived, the baby's balls were hanging out of me—it was definitely a boy! The doctor told me he would have to do an episiotomy. Then he pulled the baby's legs out and told me to push as hard as I could. With three pushes and some maneuvering, the hot, wet, bloody baby was laid on my belly. I could see his little nose flare as he breathed, then he gave a little tremolo cry that sounded like a lamb. My baby was born—a natural breech delivery. As I was wheeled back to my room, I saw on the blackboard that I had been scheduled for a c-section; I had made it by one hour.

The morning sun streamed through the window of my room and as we closed the curtains and faced our baby away from the light, he opened his eyes and looked all around. We felt so blessed. I was surprised at how good I felt, so light and bouncy. I was happy to have my body back again, but also glad to have given it up for a while to be granted this small child, so precious.

🐾     🐾     🐾

Five and a half years later we decided to increase our family. Our first child, Morgan, inherited my unusual body and legs but is a sweet and wonderful person nonetheless. We prayed to the spirits to give us another healthy child, but with strong legs. I figured that since my son was so like me, if we were to have a daughter she would be more like Wesley.

I read a book on how to determine the sex of babies and tried the suggested timing and douches. It worked great as a method of birth control. After three months, I began to wonder if everything was working all right. Then I got sick and had to take antibiotics, so we decided not to try to make a baby that month. We stopped lovemaking a week before my ovulation, but as fate would have it, I ovulated four days early and conceived anyway. We hoped that a girl spirit had come to us but were willing to accept whatever happened.

The pregnancy progressed fine. At one point I wondered if it was twins because of so much activity inside (Wesley's mother is a twin), but the doctor said there was only one heartbeat. The baby was so active I was surprised that even at such an early stage things could be so different. After Morgan's birth, I figured I could handle anything. We had moved to the country and I could have easily chosen a homebirth, but since it was a forty-five-minute drive on a winding mountain road to get to town, we decided to have the birth in a house in town that we shared with friends.

It was ten days before my due date and I was having light contractions. Around four in the afternoon I timed them and they were coming every ten minutes. By nine that night, they were still ten minutes apart, and I was tired and wanted to get some sleep. I drank some brandy, hoping that it would stop the contractions, and then went to bed. They slowed down, then picked up, but one more shot of brandy gave me a good night's rest and the energy I would need to continue the next day.

We woke early, packed the car, gathered up Morgan and his toys and headed to town. I drove most of the way rather than being bumped around as a passenger. It was breakfast time and I was starving. Fortunately my midwife, Becca, was at the restaurant and said, "Sure, eat if you're hungry. It may come up later, but do what feels right."

After breakfast I went to the Clinic and was told I was 2 centimeters dilated. We went to do laundry and by afternoon I wanted to lie in bed. Wesley took Morgan out for a little while and I was left alone in peace and quiet. Becca came over and checked me, and I was 5 centimeters. I was a little disappointed because it seemed like I should have been farther along, but she said everything was fine and that she'd come back when we called her.

Hours went by. Once again I watched my body as it did its birth dance—my belly rising and falling with each contraction. I was amazed and thrilled by how efficiently the body works if given a chance. How nice it was to be in a home setting, calm and quiet. The contractions were strong and powerful. Wesley could tell that they were taking all my concentration. We called the midwives and they came quickly, but by the time they arrived, I had gone through transition and was beginning to push. It was completely different from Morgan's birth—it was urgent. The contractions were back-to-back with no time to relax and catch my breath. The midwives had to wait about ten minutes before they could check me, but they could see right away that the baby would be born soon.

I got into a better position for delivery and Kate listened to the heartbeat. Something was wrong—the baby's heart rate was going down. She said, "Quick, push the baby out!" There went the perineal massage and the slow stretch. Ummph, I pushed and with a burning flash the head was born. The cord was wrapped tightly around the neck three times, too tightly to be pulled over the head, so it had to be cut. There was a moment of confusion before somebody found the scissors, and then, with another big push, a floppy blue baby was born.

I sat up immediately and started saying, "Come on baby, breathe! Come on baby, breathe!" The baby lay there and the midwives hovered around, slapping her feet and rubbing her back. Just as they got the oxygen up to her face, she took her first breath. I knew she would be OK. She! We had succeeded at getting a girl and she looked like she had good legs.

Morgan had been watching in wonder the whole time. He came over and we all stared at the new spirit who had come into our world—her fingernails were a henna orange, her fingers still blue but fading to pink. We all felt so grateful to the midwives and so blessed.

The birth of my daughter, Mariah, was harder on me than my first birth—perhaps it was the exertion of pushing so hard and fast. My body was tired and all I wanted to do was lie down and rest. She weighed seven and a half pounds. I thought of how energetic I had felt after Morgan's birth and wondered if it was because I had been five years younger or because the baby weighed one-and-a-half pounds less—probably both. We were delighted; our family was now complete.

*Susan divides her time between being a gardener, a house builder and a leather worker. She travels with her family to craft fairs selling their leather goods. In her spare time she enjoys spinning and needle work.*

# Clover's Journey

by Pam Wellish

---

My two year old is taking her nap on the living room floor—toys, papers, clothing are strewn about the room. The painful years of longing for her are over, and I can scarcely remember a time when she didn't exist; I feel as if I have known her all of my life.

🐚　　　🐚　　　🐚

Clover's journey into the world begins one afternoon when I am eight and a half months pregnant, and my water starts to leak. Before long it has broken fully, and my husband David and I know we have to start preparing for the arrival of a baby.

Lily is to be my midwife. Unable to reach her, and with our backup midwife out of town, we phone Kate, who is on call. I am in very early labor. There is no real need for a midwife to be with me, but I am nervous, so I ask Kate to come over.

Sitting at the dining room table, the quiet night air surrounding us, Kate listens to the baby's heartbeat. Her touch is so tender and gentle; I trust her instantly.

After a restless night, morning finally comes. Kate has gone home, and Lily has arrived with my friend Angela. We spend the day puttering about: We take a walk and fix meals I can't eat; I have an enema and then a hot shower. Every few minutes I stop to breathe with my contractions. Lily checks me in the afternoon and I am 2 centimeters dilated.

As evening settles in, my contractions grow stronger. While Lily naps, Angela rubs my feet, and David breathes with me during contractions. Angela finds a spot on my foot that, when she rubs it, makes my contractions really strong. My legs shake, and I feel like vomiting. Could this be transition, we wonder. No, I think, it's too soon (though it's been twenty-four hours).

At 11:00 p.m. Kate comes back. She checks me, and to my dismay, I am only 1½ centimeters dilated.

Lily and Kate go to the table to talk. There wouldn't be so much concern if my water sac was still intact, but it isn't. They come back and tell me they think it is time for me to go to the hospital. With broken waters the chance of infection increases. Kate thinks I will need Pitocin. They want me to make the decision, and, of course, I decide to go.

As we are preparing to leave, Kate, who isn't going with us, suggests to Lily that we take water for me to drink on the long drive. (Because our local hospital does not have a fetal heart monitor and is therefore not equipped to use Pitocin, we must go to a larger hospital, an hour and a half away.) Suddenly, the echo of words I've read in some childbirth book runs through my mind: Don't eat or drink anything if there is a possibility of a cesarean. Fear flows through me—fear of the hospital, fear of what lies ahead, fear of this awesome power to which I must surrender myself.

I try to say it casually. "Maybe I'd better not drink anything, just in case I have to have a cesarean."

Instantly Kate is kneeling by my side. "Do you think you're going to have a cesarean?" she asks, her eyes full of concern.

I am startled by the intensity of her reaction. "Well, no," I tell her. "But you never know," I add as I think of friends who have had unexpected cesareans.

She looks into my eyes and says, "Pam, you aren't going to have a cesarean." She has more faith in me than I do, and I am touched.

Finally, we are on our way. I have several strong contractions as we drive down our bumpy dirt road, but then I fall asleep, and when I awake we are there.

The brightly-lit hospital contrasts sharply with the almost pitch-dark of the night. There is an eerie feeling as we enter this quiet, glowing world. We walk past the nursery and stop to look at the tiny babies in their plastic boxes. Is this why I'm here?

I settle into a bed in the labor room. At 3:00 a.m., a nurse comes to check me—I'm 3 centimeters dilated. Everyone is relieved; I'm finally getting somewhere.

Progress is steady until morning when I get to 8 centimeters and stay there. Hours and contractions fly by. Angela sits by my side, holding my hand, looking into my eyes. We breathe slowly and deeply together. I need to—I can't do anything else.

Finally, at 11:00 a.m. I am hooked up to Pitocin and a fetal heart monitor. I can't comprehend the explanations of the numbers, graphs and blinking lights. I look up, and the monitor reads 95 for the baby's heart rate. I'm afraid that something is wrong, but no one seems concerned. I decide not to look at it any more.

At 1:00 p.m. they tell me I can push. I don't really need to, but

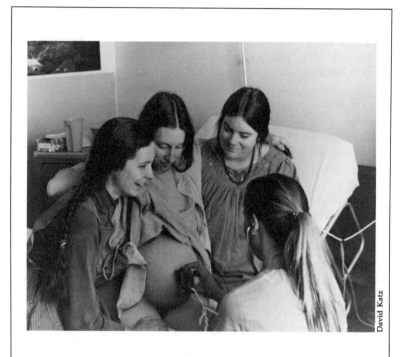

David Katz

I try it anyway. To my surprise it hurts. An hour and a half later we can see the head. The doctor, who isn't pleased about having to deliver this ill-fated homebirth attempt, comes in and sets up his table of sterile instruments. As the baby crowns I hear Lily say, "Oh, please don't cut her." He is planning to do an episiotomy without asking me. I tell him I don't want one, and he puts the syringe down. He is annoyed.

Everyone's yelling, "Push, push, you're doing good, push, push!" The room suddenly fills with nurses. I push with absolutely everything I have, and the head is out. It's 3:06 p.m. The next thing I know, the baby is being lifted onto my stomach, and the belts from the fetal heart monitor are in the way, just as Lily had warned.

"What is it?" asks a nurse. It? I think, realizing I haven't even wondered this myself. She lifts the legs apart and says, "It's a girl." A girl! I am so happy. My wish, a wish I have barely allowed myself to have, has come true. I can't believe how lucky I am.

The head came out quickly, tearing me. The doctor stitches me up, and they move me to my room. I feel very out of it. "Am I OK? Am I bleeding too much?" I ask.

"No, you're fine," they tell me.

Angela says, "Don't worry if you don't feel like holding her right away, it'll come." Who is she, this baby of mine?

Lily and Angela go home, exhausted. David falls asleep at the foot of my bed; Clover is asleep in her little plastic box. It's finally over.

        ❦        ❦        ❦

No, it was just beginning.

*Pam is currently building a home for herself and Clover. She is a peace and justice activist who is committed to civil disobedience and consequently, frequently finds herself in jail. She says, "My main priority is resistance to the forces that threaten to end life on Mother Earth. Life is sacred and I love it too much to be able to watch it being destroyed."*

# The Birth of Caitlin

by Ann Smyth Foley

August 11—It's eleven days past my due date. After a labor of over thirty hours, I finally look at my newborn daughter. She's absolutely gorgeous. I see everyone in our family in her. She's a part of all of us, and we're all a part of her, the bonding of two families.

❦          ❦          ❦

Labor was totally different from what I had expected. I spent the first part standing, which felt most natural. During contractions I'd clutch onto one of the big oaks, or put my arms around Tom, whom I called "my tree." I hadn't expected contractions to be so intense. Mine peaked very fast without much warning for a cleansing breath, but luckily they were short, and the intensity didn't last long. I don't think any Lamaze classes or reading can completely prepare you for the actual thing. I found my own totally individual way of breathing that seemed to come from some ancient place, deep down in my gut or my soul, a primordial force that I had never before tuned into: deep, deep breaths like the surging of the ocean, and an ancient language perhaps of Gaelic origin—who knows? But it all worked in keeping me going, keeping me strong through the whole thing.

I did have moments of wanting to give up: when the lip of my cervix swelled, and for hours I had to keep from pushing by blowing through every contraction. The urge to push was just too strong. I needed everyone's complete attention, eye to eye. Tom said mine were bulging out of my head.

Then pushing for hours and hours—on hands and knees, standing, or straddled over Tom's legs. Down, baby, down! You want to come out. I tried all sorts of positions to push the baby down, while Lorraine maneuvered its head and my cervix. The baby's head was presenting in an odd way, probably because that was the only way she could find to fit through my somewhat narrow pelvis.

Finally her head was through the pelvis and the cervix, moving down into my vagina. I thought, There's no way I can open up any more, there's no way that big head can come out of such a tight place. Lorraine massaged my perineum, which felt uncomfortable and exposed. Giving in to the urge to push felt much better than blowing, yet I couldn't believe that my vagina could stretch any further.

With each contraction I grunted and pushed for longer than I thought I could. The baby moved down inch by inch. Just before crowning I moved onto my back, a relief for Tom's legs. Lily and Tom were behind me for the next contraction; they raised me up, pulled my legs apart, and I pushed with everything I could muster. I could see the head. I felt an intense burning, and I was scared. Lorraine worked the big head through and suctioned the nose and mouth. With the next contraction, I gave a big push, then I panted to ease the shoulders through. "It's a girl," said Lorraine's son Devlin.

Tom and I looked at each other and said, "Our wee Caitlin." We were so happy that she'd made it into the world after so much work. A miracle had happened, with Lily and Lorraine the magicians. What a relief, no more contractions, I could finally rest.

The placenta stayed inside for three hours. There was concern that I might have to go to the hospital. I was determined to get it out at home and tried conjuring up contractions. Kate arrived in time, like a breath of fresh air, and massaged my belly. A big contraction came and the cord moved down a little. Lorraine put her hand inside and could feel the placenta, but my vagina was so swollen it was clutching onto it and wouldn't let it pass through. One really strong push, a grunt and a groan, and it plopped out. Hurrah! I felt like kissing everyone and crying. It was all over, I'd done it. We had a wee baby, Caitlin.

# *Birth*

## by Tom Foley

Caitlin is two days old today and thriving
after a thirty-five-hour labor to get her born.

Ann worked so hard to make it happen and
the midwives performed magic with the Great Mother.

Lorraine chanted: "down baby, down and out,
push that baby down . . . she wants to come out."

Ann pushed and grunted and spoke from
some ancient tongue of her agony.
We held her up, we breathed with her,
we moved her all over . . . all to get that
baby down and out.

Caitlin was twisted and presented more
of her face than head.

We opened ourselves to Caitlin and she
moved down . . . we were strong; Lily stood
by Ann like a rock foundation. All in the
tipi were tested by the Great Spirit.
Ann pushed hard and long, we expanded as
we repeated: "down baby, down and out,
open, open, relax, let go, open to the
baby . . . "

she is now open to us.

# The Birth of Erin Margaret

by Ann Smyth Foley

Our second baby was born one day before the due date after eight hours of intense labor. It moved along so smoothly compared to Caitlin's birth that at moments I couldn't believe it. I felt much more prepared for this birth. I'd been through it once and knew what to expect. It was more like getting ready for a party. Both Lily and Lorraine had come out to visit, and I knew that they'd be here once again for me. My mother arrived unexpectedly from New York; she came walking down our driveway in a rainstorm. I wasn't surprised but felt really glad to see her.

Halloween day I had steady Braxton-Hicks contractions, and I knew something was happening. At 3:00 p.m. I was sitting on the edge of the bed reading over the signs of the onset of labor. I felt a contraction and then pressure, followed by a warm gush of water. What a surprise! I was very excited and happy and called to Tom and my mum to tell them the news.

Tom called Lorraine and she came right over, thinking that things would start happening soon. In the morning, after an uneventful night, Lorraine checked me: I was 2 centimeters dilated and the bag of water had sealed back up. False alarm. She left for a gathering of midwives which was happening up the road from us and said she'd be back at lunchtime.

The day continued with steady Braxton-Hicks, but nothing I had to stop and breathe for. Tom and I walked, up the road and back, down the road and back. Mum watched Caitlin. I felt very discouraged thinking this was going to be another difficult labor, with nothing happening as it should.

Our neighbors walked over to invite Caitlin to their house. She was so eager to be off with them that I could hardly get a "goodbye" in. As soon as they'd left, about 4:00 p.m., we sat down to have a cup of tea, and all of a sudden the baby started kicking like crazy. It really wanted to get out. Mum was busy cooking a big pot of mince and totties (a traditional Scottish feast), and Tom and I were upstairs breathing slowly and steadily with the contractions coming ten, eight, then five minutes apart.

The contractions got more intense after a relaxing foot bath, so we decided that it was time for Tom to run to the neighbors' to call Lorraine and that I would lie on my side to slow things down. I found lying on my side just as intense—standing was more comfortable. Tom was my "tree" once again as he had been at Caitlin's birth. While he was away, I leaned on the walls.

He returned after what seemed like ages. Lorraine arrived in no time and I was glad to see her. I was also happy and excited because I knew that this experience was going to be a lot easier and smoother. I was 4 centimeters dilated and opening. Yippee! As Lorraine scurried around sorting out birth supplies, chatting with my mum and drinking tea, Tom and I were upstairs dealing with the contractions, breathing deeply and slowly. Lily arrived.

I was upright through most of the labor, either standing or kneeling on the edge of the bed—that's what felt and worked the best. I really had to be on top of the breathing, or I'd lose it. Some contractions were much stronger than others, and I'd hyperventilate through the most intense peaks and have to hold on to Tom's hand cupped over my mouth as I breathed. That was scary, but I knew it would pass.

I reached a point where deep breathing no longer worked. I

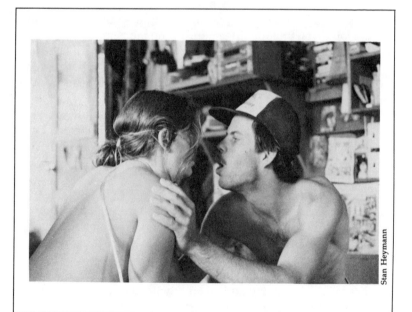

Stan Heymann

called out for help. Lily and Lorraine came up and took over for Tom. I remembered reaching that same point with Caitlin, and I had a sense of déjà vu. It was time to change to three pants and blow with a deep cleansing breath.

Lorraine brought me some broth which I sipped slowly through a straw while lying on my side. No sooner had I eaten than I threw it all up, which felt good. Then the contractions came on stronger. Lorraine checked me—8 centimeters.

Up on my feet again. There was strong back pain as the head moved down through my pelvis. I moved on to my knees, leaning my elbows and head on the bed. The midwives massaged and put pressure on my back. Gradually, with each intense peak, the pain moved farther and farther down my spine as the baby's head moved down. Swaying my hips felt good. I chanted from the bowels of my being, "Down, down!" We all chanted together.

Lorraine checked me again. The baby's head was through my cervix. I immediately asked, "Where's the swollen lip?" We all laughed. I couldn't believe there were no complications, and I was pleased with my body's ability to work so well. It was exciting, and I was exhausted. At 11:00 p.m., it was time for serious pushing. Caitlin returned and Mum kept her occupied downstairs.

I was propped up on big pillows on the bed, all set to push. I could feel the baby's head moving from side to side within me. But all of a sudden the contractions slowed down. I just wanted to rest, let the force of the contractions do the work. I sensed that Lily and Lorraine were anxious for the birth, and that made me sink more into the feeling, in my stubborn Taurus way. I wanted to take my time, this was my creation. But the baby wasn't moving and we weren't really getting anywhere, so I agreed, reluctantly, to stand up again. I was afraid deep inside that I couldn't go through with this last leg of the journey, that I didn't have energy enough to deal with that tremendous pressure.

With the next contraction I stopped thinking, squatted, and put my all behind that pushing urge, and I could feel the head bulging out from between my legs. What an uncomfortable, vulnerable feeling as I was helped back onto the bed (Tom said we were all taking teeny, tiny steps). Tremendous burning: the head emerged, cord wrapped around the neck, struggling for air. Lorraine said seriously, "You have to get the baby out, quick. Push with all your might. Now!" I did. Lorraine slipped the cord over the head and Tom caught her. In the next second she was on my belly, limp and pale. As we massaged her, she came to life and cried a hearty cry. I couldn't believe we had another girl.

Caitlin was in awe; she and my mum had watched the birth. I cut the cord, and my mum held Erin as we worked on getting the placenta out. It felt very special to have my mum there. And how could I ever thank Lily and Lorraine—I could only glow with gratitude.

# Erin's Birth

## by Tom Foley

False start Saturday afternoon, partial breaking of the waters. We called Lorraine, and she stayed the night. But it didn't happen; instead, doubts and fears about another long labor. No! We concentrated on the new baby together.

In the afternoon, our neighbors took Caitlin over to their place. We were unsure whether we wanted Caitlin to stay through the birth. It turned out to be a relief to have her away during labor so we could focus on the new baby. Sunday at 5:00 p.m., we soaked Ann's feet and strong contractions followed. I called Lorraine immediately.

❦     ❦     ❦

Contractions are intense and make Ann lean on me. She shows me how she wants me to be her "leaning tree." She's breathing deeply; I'm near her face breathing with her. She's closing her eyes, and I tell her to open them. She chides me to be quiet. I grumble but realize she's conserving strength. It's her trip.

Her arms around my shoulders pull me down, her legs tremble; we change positions. She's on the bed lying on her side when Lorraine comes and checks her: 4 centimeters. Lily comes a little later. The midwives talk downstairs while upstairs, things are getting rough. Ann calls out for help: "I'm afraid!" The midwives help her relax with massage and get her to stand up. She's moaning and panting while the baby is coming down. Lorraine leads our chant, "Down, down."

At 8 centimeters Ann says, "Where's the fat lip?" We laugh. Caitlin had been stuck on the lip of the cervix for eight hours. Ann seems disbelieving but happy. The contractions begin to come harder, and her breathing changes, her eyes reaching out desperately. The midwives tell her to sink into the contractions and keep the moaning low and deep. Ann grabs me as she buckles under; I hold her. We notice it's about 11:30 p.m., and I wonder what day the baby will be born. Ann's mom takes care of Caitlin downstairs. She's had the downstairs watch: boiling water and such. An angel!

Contractions slow down. Ann's moaning becomes low; it seems to come from some deep, ancient place. We try another position; she had been lying on me, and my back was hurting. We help her up and then have to move her to the bed again almost immediately because the baby's head pops through. We take small steps, supporting Ann and the baby's head.

I see a bluish-pink head emerge as Ann pushes. But then the contractions stop, and Ann can't seem to push. The baby is turning dark blue and gasping. Lorraine tells her, "Push, you have to push right now—the baby needs to come out." Her tone and her eye contact with Ann are serious. Ann's eyes seem to become fixed as she pushes on the next contraction. The baby's head comes out far enough for Lily to suction the nose as Lorraine pulls the cord from around the neck. The pinkish color returns as I massage the body, and I am the one to fully hold the baby and lift her onto her mother's belly.

I feel relief and gratitude to all the helpers. Everyone seems to be glowing like the kerosene lanterns. Caitlin and Ann's mom had come upstairs just before the crowning—they both look like they have experienced a miracle. Ann tells all with her tired yet rosy look. She asks Lorraine, "What is it?"

"A girl," replies Lorraine.

"Oh no!" says Ann.

We all laugh again. I call her Erin immediately, but Ann isn't so sure; she wanted a boy. Ann puts Erin to her breast, and Caitlin cries out, "My titty!" We explain about sharing once again, and Caitlin seems to accept Erin's sucking and even begins to smile.

Erin was born at 12:16 a.m., November 2. It's hard to believe this is only the beginning.

*Ann, raised in Scotland, came to the United States at an early age. She works at a local day care center, gardens, plays pennywhistle, knits, sews and makes pottery. Tom has a BA in Psychology and worked in the mental health field for five years before moving to the country. Besides being a father, a husband and a homesteader, he works for the Head Start Program, which keeps him busy. He enjoys singing, playing guitar, softball and basketball.*

# Meaghann Mariah's Birth

by Holly Nimen

---

Dear Meaghann:

Two days before your birth we went to the ocean with some friends. After being buried in the sand, I felt a gush and realizing my water had broken, I exclaimed, "Look, there's $H_2O$ coming out!" So we returned to town and stopped at the Clinic. The midwives examined me and told me that I was in early labor and that your head hadn't engaged yet. We then went home to prepare for your entrance into this world.

Our midwives, Lorraine, Kathleen and Lily, arrived at 10:00 p.m. It was a long night with lots of contractions, but when morning arrived, you still hadn't engaged. A walk was in order. It was a beautiful walk through the fog-filled meadow to the pond. We stopped every second step to breathe and chant, "Open, open." What a wonderful circle of energy! When we returned, I was 4 centimeters dilated—even 6 centimeters during a contraction. But your head *still* hadn't engaged.

There was some concern because the water had broken and you were not coming down. Questions started to arise. By noon Lorraine felt something needed to be done, so she called Dr. Bill. My greatest fear was having to go to a distant hospital, to some strange doctors, and to who knows what. But Dr. Bill said to come to the local hospital and he'd help us. We discovered forewaters and we hoped that breaking them would mean a quick descent into the world for you.

We arrived at the hospital at 5:00 p.m. With a quick rush and stir the forewaters were broken but to no avail. You wouldn't budge. So again, more waiting, more contractions, and much more concern. It had been twenty-four hours since the waters had first broken, and the risk of infection was increasing. What to do? A cesarean section was being discussed. Why me? It hadn't been my fear or even once a thought. But the decision was made; it had been too long without your head engaging.

There we all were, me exhausted and all the ladies saddened. Had modern medicine suddenly taken over? Was there really no

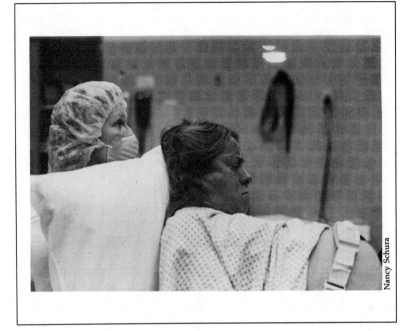

Nancy Schura

way you were going to come out?

I was sent to x-ray. They said I was too narrow from front to back, and you were presenting at the wrong angle. They prepped me: IV, catheter and shave. Thank goodness they gave me a shot of Nisentil, because at that point I left this world; it was too much. But the thought of you being born in two hours was a relief.

Dr. Bill came in after I was prepped, and by some miracle, Meaghann, you moved. Just a little, but you moved—through the hope and prayers of all those wonderful ladies who had bonded for you and your birth. Bill gave us another forty-five minutes to see what would happen.

I rested and I walked—lo and behold you moved down more. Thank you Lord! The c-section was put on hold. All I asked for was some rest. I remember sleeping through contractions and every now and then being woken by a strong one. By morning you had finally engaged, and I was fully dilated, forty hours after the waters had broken.

Now the real work—pushing. Four hours of it, in every position, and with everyone involved. Lorraine manually turned you because of your presentation. What a feeling, what a sensation, what a lot of work. And of course you and I moved slowly.

There was a time when I was almost willing to try anything to get you out. How about forceps? I felt badly giving up at that point, and worse because Dr. Bill came in and was ready to use them, anything to help me. I guess his desire to take care of us became pretty strong. But I kept pushing. Soon we saw the top of your head, a bluish-purple circle. At first you kept ducking back, but soon you stayed. Finally, with Dr. Bill opening one side of the perineum and me holding the other, you crowned. Your crowning was quick: another push, maybe two, and you were out with open eyes. I asked, "What is it?"

"A girl," Lily said.

I shouted, "Thank God!" Meaghann Mariah had been born.

You were too quick for Dr. Bill. You cried before he could get all the fluid out of your mouth, so a little got in your lungs. It made your breathing a bit fast, but everything was OK. We put tetracycline drops in your eyes and gave you a shot of vitamin K.

A friend stayed with us that night in the hospital. You spent some time in her arms since I was so tired. The next morning Dr. Bill came and told us everything was fine, so we were homeward bound. The rest of the story is just us getting used to each other. Happy birth.

Love, Mom

*Holly chose to have Meaghann without a partner and is a single parent. She and Meaghann live in a rural town where she grows much of her own food. She works part-time at a food co-op and is involved in ecological activism, working in a local campaign against mandatory insecticide spraying. She enjoys tennis, volleyball and swimming.*

# Pablo

by Cecelia Rahner

It has been four and a half years since my son Pablo was born. Throughout my pregnancy I was healthy, physically and emotionally, but I was put into the "high risk" category because of a previous stillbirth.

Various blood tests revealed that my placenta was functioning at a very minimal level, so I went into the hospital for closer scrutiny. It was during this time that Pablo was born, two and a half weeks early.

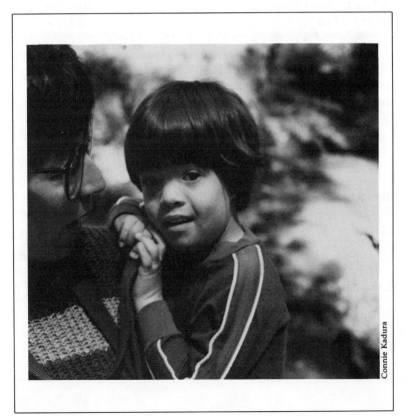

Connie Kadura

My husband, my breathing coach, my midwife, my obstetrician and a pediatrician were all present at the birth, so I had lots of support. As my labor lasted two full days, everyone was indispensable.

At birth, Pablo's condition was poor. His ability to maintain his body temperature was faulty, but his lungs seemed sound. We spent a week stabilizing before going home. A week later, we were back in the hospital, this time on an emergency basis. Hypothermia seemed to be only a symptom of Pablo's problem. The doctors discussed various possible causes with us. Perhaps he had some unidentified virus, or maybe his thyroid wasn't functioning properly, and finally a chromosomal abnormality was suggested as a possible answer. He was treated with antibiotics and put into an isolette for another week. I was thankful that I could room-in with him, touch him and nurse him.

It wasn't until months later that we were told the results of Pablo's blood tests: he had Down's syndrome. This condition is a chromosomal abnormality which develops at fertilization. An extra chromosome containing thousands of genes appears in the baby's first cell. This error in cell division continues as the baby develops so that there are forty-seven instead of forty-six chromosomes in most or all of the body cells. The end result of this imbalance is a group of symptoms, of which mental retardation is one.

I reacted to this somewhat hysterically at first, but after tears and sorrow, and with the support of my husband, I settled down and saw the reality of our sweet, responsive and loving son. We anticipated that we would have to do much more for him to help him achieve his full potential, but so far it's made parenting much more complete. His happy, loving spirit fills our days with joy and hope.

*Cecilia has moved to a city where Pablo attends a school for exceptional children. She works as an aide at his school and hopes to further her education, specializing in speech therapy.*

# By the Light
# of the Moon

by Kathi Chandler

---

So there's a baby within me—incredible! It's been living there for nine weeks already; I don't feel it, and I can't see it bulging out my belly yet, but I do feel quite magical.

Chris and I have a busy summer ahead of us, with lots of work to do. We live in a small bus, which is fine for us, but now with a child coming we'll need more room. Chris has drawn up a beautiful houseplan. It will be a fine home for us on top of our mountain. As soon as the rains quit, we can begin.

❦    ❦    ❦

Construction is under way. Our neighbor and Chris' father come to help. My belly is growing by now, but I do what I can. Long, busy summer days. Being pregnant is not long naps and sunning away the hours down by the river, at least not this time. We've got a house to build.

❦    ❦    ❦

The pressure is building; due day is Saturday. The house just isn't ready yet—sawdust, piles of lumber, general construction chaos right in the room where we plan to birth our child. We go to sleep each evening with visions of a middle-of-the-night hurried sweep to clear a corner for our birth.

Then to the rescue, father and friends—all pitch in. By Saturday the house is done. Due day, moving day. In come the furniture, bed and rugs, and at last I can unpack our baby's things. Sigh of relief.

Busy day, early to bed, first night in our new bedroom. Chris is asleep; I'm lying awake gazing out at the stars, feeling very content, in my nest at last.

❦    ❦    ❦

I think a ready state of mind has a lot to do with the onset of labor because just then, labor began. I had been having light contractions for several days, but this was different. I lay there for a while feeling thrilled, then I thought about what a mess my kitchen was, and about the sandwich spread I had intended to make for the midwives and friends who were to be present. So, with a burst of energy, I slipped downstairs, cleaned up and made the sandwich spread, stopping to breathe through contractions. Two hours later I went back to bed.

Contractions let up after a while, and I got about an hour and a half of sleep before they came back, harder this time. Chris awoke to my blowing and puffing around 2:00 a.m. and asked, "How long has this been going on?"

"Since ten o'clock," I told him. He was wide awake instantly and began timing my contractions.

After two hours of regular and increasingly frequent contractions, we called Kate and told her not to hurry, but things were in motion. About two hours later, at 6:00 a.m., the phone rang. Kate had run low on gas trying to find our road and wasn't sure she could make it up the mountain. So Chris went down to get her. I lay there alone in the lantern light, listening to music, feeling dreamy and strong, breathing through my contractions all alone.

Soon Chris and Kate were back, and the arrival of our midwife brought a halt to my contractions. Nothing—a complete stop. How embarrassing! Kate went out to our old home, the bus, and slept until 9:00 a.m. I slept too, while Chris stayed wide awake. By noon there wasn't much more than an occasional contraction. I was 2½ centimeters dilated. Kate decided to go home until things picked up. Chris drove her down to her car at the bottom of the mountain. As I heard them leave, the contractions came on again and stayed. When Chris returned, the contractions were quite regular. We sat together for a long time, feeling close. Then the friends we had invited to be at the birth arrived.

I decided a hot bath would be nice. After about an hour of labor in the tub, I was feeling relaxed. Chris helped me back to bed and then called Kate. In forty-five minutes she was back. I was 8 centimeters dilated and it was 4:00 p.m.

Another friend who had been giving me energy treatments called "Jin Shin Jyutsu" during my pregnancy joined us. She gave me a treatment, Chris rubbed my back, and another friend braided my hair—all those loving hands certainly were appreciated.

By 6:00 p.m. I was fully dilated. It was time to push. It had been hard to refrain from pushing during the last contractions. Chris and I had been present at a birth where four short pushes were all it took to get the baby out. I was expecting the same, but that was not to be for me. Almost two hours of constant pushing with short breaks in between didn't bring us our baby. Lying on my side, squatting, sitting up, standing, or to be more precise, hanging from Chris' and Kate's shoulders as they stood—pushing, pushing. Whew, hard work!

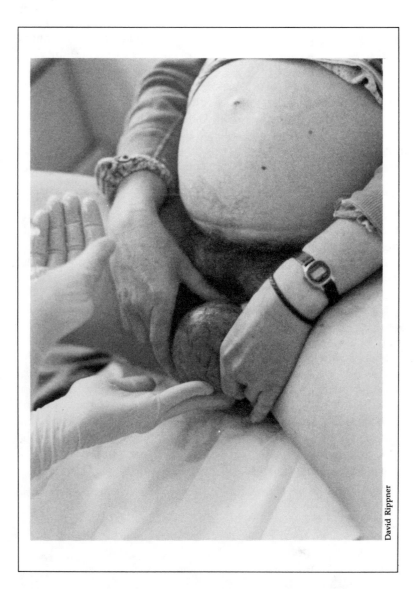

David Rippner

It was after 7:30 p.m.; the moon and stars were out. Chris and I went outside on our deck where we had rigged up a bucket with a toilet seat—it felt like a royal throne. Now *there* was a familiar and comfortable position. It took only three more contractions and some "howling at the moon good pushes," and I could feel the head move down. I'm sure I calmly said, "Chris, I feel the baby coming." But Chris says that isn't quite the way it was. He could tell something was happening, though. He picked up his flashlight and took a peek, and that was his first look at our daughter.

Chris and the midwives got me back inside on my bed. As they were getting ready for the next set of contractions, setting up a sterile field, etc., my muscles pulled the baby back inside. I thought, Damn, all that work and she goes sliding away again. But the next contraction brought her right back. Chris got a mirror so I could see our baby too. That really let me know just how close I was to having her. She was right there, lots of hair. I touched her. All my exhaustion left me and was replaced by excitement.

"Push! Hold! Ease her out! We waited this long, we can wait a few minutes more to keep you from tearing," said Kate. With the help of the mirror, which Chris was holding at just the right angle despite his excitement, I could see how much I was moving her and if I was keeping her from slipping back between contractions. There was the burning feeling I was told about, but it wasn't bad. At that point nothing mattered except that I was moments away from seeing my baby. Then there it was, the whole head. Kate went to work suctioning the mouth and nose, waiting for the next contraction. Then it came, bringing out the body. Such a relief, such a wonderful feeling.

Friends circled close, Chris by my side, all of us staring in wonder at the gorgeous little creature lying there in the lantern light. She was so relaxed, so mellow, just stretching and sighing and blinking. They laid her on my belly, and when the pulsing stopped, Chris cut the cord. Welcome to this world, little one. She was wrapped in a blanket, and I took her to my breast. Our baby, our daughter, a product of our love, so beautiful.

*Kathi and her family have recently moved to a small town near the ocean in the Santa Cruz Mountains. She writes, "Cali is a great kid, the pride and joy of her mom and dad."*

# Full Circle

by Rosie Bosco

My first pregnancy was a rough one: I was anemic, overweight and tired when my waters broke early on the morning of my thirty-first birthday. Contractions started very slowly. I was so excited I couldn't sit still. In the afternoon my husband Willie and I went shopping, and the ride on the dirt road sped things up. By 5:00 p.m. the contractions were getting stronger and more regular. We called our midwives, Kate and Kathleen, and settled in for our home delivery.

Well, things didn't go exactly as we'd planned. The place I'd prepared for a birthing platform turned out to be terribly uncomfortable. I couldn't figure out how to lie down, so I paced a lot and squatted during the most intense pains. My coaches did everything imaginable. We tried different positions, different breathing patterns and different focus points, but we never seemed to find the key to getting me into it. I kept fighting it.

By 2:00 a.m. I was only 2 centimeters dilated and already totally exhausted. I was also freaked out. The experience was very psychedelic. My beautiful, comfortable home turned into a cluttered, busy, badly-lit, uncomfortable trap. The people I loved turned into frightening, disembodied, floating eyeballs, noses and mouths. Their voices became accusing, and I felt paranoid and isolated. I remember screaming, "Get me out of here!"—out of the room, out of the pain, out of the whole miserable situation.

By dawn I was fully dilated, but had developed an anterior cervical lip. Each check was agony. Finally, it was time to push. So I pushed. And pushed. And pushed. Nothing happened. I couldn't feel any urges; I couldn't feel the baby. Hours passed, and I started getting hysterical. I was shaking and crying and didn't understand what was wrong. When Kate suggested that we go to the hospital, I was shocked. *What? Me give up?* I thought. Then, *You mean there's an alternative to this?* And finally, *Sure, let's go.* I was having trouble thinking and talking. I hadn't smiled for hours. I was really glad something was going to change.

When we arrived at the hospital, Dr. Bill appeared to me as an angel with glowing white light around his head. I really was hallucinating! He had come to deliver me from this horrible night-mare.

I was taken to the labor room where I was given a shot to relax me, and Dr. Bill tried to get me to push the baby out. He showed me the head in a mirror and gave me lots of encouragement, but no luck. She just didn't want to come, and I couldn't push any more. I was tired of the pain, tired of pushing, and was ready to give up and die. My contractions had almost completely stopped, and they were so far apart they weren't doing any good anyway. The baby would come down a little bit, then go right back. No progress.

Then I was taken into the delivery room for a forceps delivery. No drugs: I had to "be there" to help push her out. Dr. Bill gave me Novacain for the episiotomy, then went to work. I never saw or felt the baby. All I was aware of was the pain: horrible, excruciating pain, and the sound of my screaming. Willie had to tell me the baby was out.

She was gorgeous, of course—eight pounds, fourteen ounces and built like a bunch of sausages. They gave me gas while they stitched me up. I was so happy to see Laura-Jo. I fell in love with her immediately. She was strong throughout the ordeal; she never showed any signs of distress. She had a big bloody mark on her face from the forceps, but it didn't seem to bother her.

I cried for three days. I felt so gypped. There went my hopes for the perfect lotus-flower-opening homebirth I'd set my heart on.

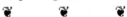

When I became pregnant with my second child, I decided not to try another homebirth, and we made arrangements for a hospital delivery.

One day toward the end of my pregnancy, as I was doing a birth visualization in the prenatal yoga class, all the memories of my first birth came rushing back. I realized I was terrified of giving birth again. I sobbed uncontrollably while everyone comforted me. Kathleen came over to my house that weekend, and we re-did the imagery. Instead of fear, anger, pain, self-pity and failure, I concentrated on giving all the responsibility to God. I decided to let Him control the event, and all my negative images changed to those of strength, power and success. With Kathleen's encouragement and suggestions, I realized that if I let God take care of me, through the strength that my faith in Jesus Christ had given me, I wouldn't have to be afraid.

Things went differently this time. Giving birth a second time was less scary because I knew what to expect—there weren't as many surprises.

My labor began at 1:00 p.m. We calmly packed up and drove to town; I was "calm" because I'd had four false labors and I'd been ready for months. We dropped off Laura-Jo and Willie's son, Vito, visited an art show, then went to see Kathleen. She said I was 2 centimeters dilated and suggested we go to a motel near the hospital to wait until things started getting more intense—she was going to see a movie. After the long labor I'd had the first time, we were expecting this one to take a while to get started.

We went to a motel, and the manager, having no rooms, offered us her apartment. We went to see it, and it was lovely, but then I got an uncomfortable feeling and knew it was time to settle into a permanent nest. I felt that once I got settled, I wouldn't want to move again. So we decided to go straight to the hospital.

Once we got there, things went like clockwork. Kathleen came by, and I was having good, strong contractions, so she decided to stay with me. She helped me take a bath, put my things away and get into my nightgown. Willie brought me a fruit salad and we started watching TV. The atmosphere was nice and cozy.

Things went really well. Another midwife, Mary, came to help at 7:00 p.m., and by 9:00, Dr. Bill was there. We turned off the TV when I started seeing the colors blur and move from the screen to the walls. From then on it was serious business. Kathleen got me to lower my voice and "get down in the pain." None of that fancy breathing worked this time; I was groaning like an animal. It was hard, but I kept praying to God, and by 10:00 p.m. I was 7 centimeters dilated.

When it was time to push, I knew it and gave it everything I had. It was great to have something to do with all that pain instead of just having to ride it; "riding" contractions is like trying to remain calm and uninvolved while a tiger slowly eats your foot. It was so fantastic to have the power to push. I wasn't exhausted from a long first stage and I felt like Wonder Woman.

In five big pushes, Ruth Ella was born. I actually felt her leave my body and slide out. No tears, no cuts, no stitches. Instead of feeling sorry for myself, I was proud, especially since she'd come out face up ("sunny-side up"), and I'd had to endure an extra intense back labor because of her position.

I felt fulfilled and satisfied. I had come full circle. Now I know what a normal birth is, and I thank God for giving me the opportunity to deliver this way, the way I wanted it to be. I had two very different births, and now I have two perfect daughters.

*Rosie has been a musician all her life and studied North Indian classical music for eight years with Ali Akbar Khan. She is well-known in the community as a sitar player. She says, "I feel blessed with the full-time task of teaching and raising the two children God has given me and my husband, and I am growing in my knowledge of Jesus Christ. I hope to be able to someday use my experience, my music, my training, indeed my whole being, in the service of the Lord."*

# A Midwife Gives Birth

by Lily and Stan

*Stan:* Lily was three days past her due date and she was huge. Everything was ready. We expected my parents to arrive in three days for their first visit. Would our baby arrive before they did? We went to town hoping that the ride on the long bumpy road would get things going.

*Lily:* Sure enough, after dinner I started feeling real contractions. We went to bed early. I dozed a couple of hours and woke around midnight feeling low pressure with contractions ten to fifteen minutes apart. I decided to ignore them and lay in bed with my watch, my hot water bottle and my thoughts. I was up every hour until dawn emptying my bowels. A lovely pink sunrise greeted the day.

*Stan:* I was very excited—our babe would be born today. I checked Lily and she was 3 centimeters dilated. We decided to send our son Journey to school. A neighbor would bring him home early if the baby came faster than we expected.

*Lily:* After Stan checked my cervix, I knew I was really in labor, but because my previous births had been so long and exhausting, I didn't want to give it much energy. Going about my daily routine helped distract me. Stan was busy outside gathering firewood.

*Stan:* I was around the house, always within hearing distance of Lily's labor sounds. A friend dropped by and carried our daughter Chamisa, who was not yet two years old, for a walk through our gardens; she was soon asleep.

*Lily:* Stan and I had a couple of nice hours together, our only time alone during the labor. We sat in front of the fire, teary-eyed, sharing our feelings—time seemed to stop. It was new for me to have a labor that progressed quickly. This time, my final birth, I was determined to have fun!

*Stan:* At noon Lily was 5 centimeters dilated and having rushes five minutes apart. We had thought that the baby was breech but now we could tell that it was the head that was presenting. Chamisa woke from her nap and Journey returned from school. Rebecca, who was going to assist with the birth, arrived with her partner, Proud.

*Lily:* At four o'clock I was 8 centimeters dilated and Becca reassured me that everything was fine and moving quickly. Having supportive and loving friends was comforting as the contractions became very close and heavy—it felt like a lot of work to me.

*Stan:* The contractions grew stronger as afternoon faded into evening. Lily had a bath. Now she was 9 centimeters dilated and the pressure was intense so she had Becca break the bag of waters. After a few more contractions, gushes of water came out, stained slightly green.

*Lily:* I was feeling disheartened and wimpy. I insisted that Stan draw another bath, although he thought it would only slow me down. I got in and the minute my bottom hit the water, I had to push. I began pushing and there was no way I could stop. I tried pushing while sitting in the bathtub, but that didn't feel right. Neither did squatting in the water. I remember feeling almost frantic at this point. I could push with these contractions, which reduced the feeling of pain and pressure and made me feel like I was doing something instead of being carried by the contractions— yet pushing was so intense, so heavy, I wasn't sure if I could do it. I got out of the water and had a few more contractions on the birthing seat.

*Stan:* I supported Lily's vagina while she pushed, all the time telling her that the baby was moving down. She wasn't easily convinced but kept pushing harder and harder.

*Lily:* I felt up inside myself and couldn't feel the baby's head. I was discouraged—my pushing wasn't moving the baby.

*Stan:* We moved to the bed and Lily gave it her all. On her knees, facing me, she pushed with incredible strength.

*Lily:* Suddenly I yelled to Rebecca, "It's burning! Quick Rebecca, it's burning!" Immediately she told me to blow. Stan was blowing with me. I tried my hardest to blow, though my body wanted so much to push. Rebecca helped me turn over to a semi-sitting position so I could participate.

*Stan:* There was a whirlwind of activity around us. Lily kept me with her, face to face, reminding her to blow and relax. Everyone was hurrying into the bedroom. The sounds told them, This is it!

As I supported Lily's vagina with my hand, Rebecca managed to apply some olive oil. A few more pushes and the baby's head was crowning.

*Lily:* I was confused when Rebecca asked me to push again because it felt like the head had been born. With another push the head was all the way out and Becca slipped the cord from around the baby's neck. I reached down and felt a large wet head between my legs.

*Stan:* At this point Chamisa became upset. I took her on my knee and comforted her. Although I had hoped to catch this baby, it was obvious that Rebecca would have to help instead. The shoulders were not coming. Lily had no more contractions, but Rebecca told her to push anyway as she put traction on the head. I could see that it wasn't working, so I told Lily to get up. In a squatting position, with support from Proud, she pushed the baby right out.

*Lily:* It felt so hard to change positions, but I knew I had to be up to push this big baby out. Pushing hard, I felt the body slip down and out of my birth canal, landing on the bed. It was 8:44 p.m. Immediately I looked down and saw that we had another daughter. Oh good! I reached over and scooped her up into my loving arms. After a few rubs and a whiff of oxygen, she cried and looked around. Although she was a little floppy, she pinked up quickly. I felt overwhelmed with thankfulness and joy. Such a beautiful, healthy girl. When the long umbilical cord stopped pulsating, Rebecca clamped it and Journey had the honor of cutting his sister free. I felt a strong contraction and knew the placenta was ready to come out. I handed the baby to Stan, squatted over a bowl, and pushed out a large intact placenta. Whew, it felt like pushing out a small baby!

*Stan:* Anna Rose gazed at her mother. Smiling faces surrounded her—I was delighted. Mixed with joy were the thrill and relief of being witness to one of the supreme transitions shared by all humanity. With this passage comes the innate sense of purpose and self-confidence which is each person's birthright. As parents and birth attendants, we are here to receive the newborn with love and guidance.

*Lily:* As friends cleaned up, I took a shower, feeling great. Stan and Rebecca were weighing the baby as I walked back to the bedroom. Seeing the scale pass ten pounds, I leaned on Proud's shoulder in

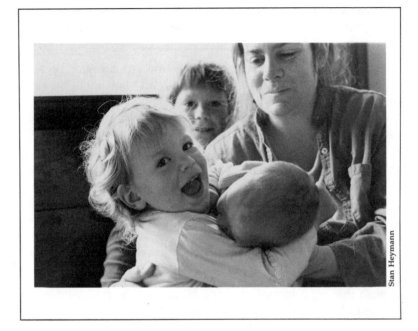

Stan Heymann

near disbelief—a ten-and-a-half-pound baby and I didn't tear! Settling down to nurse my new baby with my family all around, I was ready for a good night's sleep. Such precious moments.

🐚    🐚    🐚

I am often asked if being a midwife has influenced the way I give birth. Really, very little—I am still a woman in an emotionally and physically vulnerable place who needs the support and love of my mate and friends. I need the reassurance of someone telling me I'm doing fine and that the pain is not going to continue forever. Of course, being so familiar with the birth process gives me confidence; my body knows how to birth as long as I surrender and let it happen. I have learned a lot from my recent pregnancies and births and now have a deeper understanding as a midwife. I feel a stronger empathy with the women I help; now I know how hard it is to do some of the things I have asked women to do in labor. I feel so blessed to have given birth to three beautiful, healthy children at home.

# *This Light*
## by Lily

*light upon my path*
*closing eyes to feel clearer*
*pushing hard to make it come*
*sweat*
*smell of incense*
*sounds of music, people*
*distant—not of me.*
*this labor,*
*these waves of chilling force*
*and this hand, tightly linked with mine,*
*are my only realities*
*and I am absorbed.*
*with wonder, gazing, holding,*
*feeling this sudden life born of me*
*this is the first moment I really understand*
*what it is we have created and asked blessing for*
*and I am indeed thankful for this light.*

*Lily and Stan live on their ninety-four acre homestead, Filaree Farm, where they raise vegetables, orchard fruit and angora rabbits. Lily has been involved with midwifery since the birth of her son, Journey, eleven years ago. Stan has attended and photographed many homebirths and says it has deepened his perspective and appreciation of women and children.*

# From Dark to Light

by Dianne Magnatta

---

It was a different type of day—I awoke feeling tingly. A thick bloody discharge was falling from my widening cervix, and the contractions I had experienced since mid-September had a new-ness to them. Could this be the day? Yes, I was sure. Should I tell Thom? He would get excited, and what if I was wrong? I decided to wait. Thom sat eating huge cloves of garlic. The scent of garlic while I was pregnant was sure to bring on nausea. The need for fresh air overwhelmed me so I suggested we go to town to see what the discharge meant.

Kathleen, the midwife who would be attending my birth, saw me in the Clinic. (We had just had dinner together the night before.) She was calm about my new condition and said that the birth could be in a few hours or a few days. The contractions seemed deeper, yet were still gentle. My emotions seemed touchy, and the world had a different glow about it, almost a golden shimmer.

Then suddenly I had a *very* different contraction—my face flushed and I leaned over. This must be the *real* contraction! So we headed to our friends' home where we planned to have the birth of our baby boy (a sonogram had shown two cute testicles and a penis).

The next ten minutes were rather surreal. I had another much more intense contraction. It hit every nerve in my body; I was surprised at the sharpness of the pain. Thom was starting to get nervous, excited and practical, all at the same time. He said, "Breathe!" Whoosh, whoosh, whoosh—big jet streams of garlic-breath were hitting me as we drove in a closed car through the redwood forest. The pain and garlic were too much for me, and I started to tell him, *Take me to the hospital now! Don't breathe on me, please!* Then the feeling subsided and I thought, This must be transition. Everything I had read suggested that at this time, some women want to go to the hospital or want medication for relief. TRANSITION! After two contractions? The excitement got to me too, and I was ecstatic. Thom rolled down his window and breathed his practiced breathing out to the forest while we drove the next two miles. I'm sure the breathing kept him very calm and under control. The next contraction was different, and I could feel movement high in my vagina. I wanted to get there fast.

When we arrived at the house, the four men who live on the land were there. Thom ran me a bath; Pepe called the midwife from a neighbor's phone; Kirsh washed the windows in the room; and Leib set up the bed: a beautiful welcome for the new boy on the land.

I found if I bent over forward, the sharpness of the contractions wasn't so intense. I leaned forward and when the bath was ready, I crawled on all fours to the tub, climbed in and stayed there on my hands and knees. The bathtub was wonderful. Kathleen had mentioned that a tub of warm water was relaxing for a laboring woman. Oh, how right she was!

I could feel the baby descending through the birth canal with each contraction. The contractions had changed. The four sharp ones were replaced with deep rhythmic periods of intense movement and release—no pain! The wonder of the womb as it comes to life to do its work, then rests again until the next child's time to be brought to our earth. Woman, womb, birth: The power of it all had me entrapped, joyfully.

The men were still busying themselves in preparation and my friend Linda was at my side. I told her the baby was at the middle of the birth canal. We were ready to deliver him together if Kathleen didn't arrive in time. All was well; there were good friends and hot water, and my body was doing its work smoothly and powerfully. I trusted myself very much.

When Kathleen came she was surprised to see how fast I had progressed in the few hours since she had last seen me. She checked me and sure enough, the baby was almost ready to be held in our arms. Kathleen got me out of my wonderful bathtub and into the birthing room, which was sparkling clean and lit with candles—good work, gentlemen! I went to the hands and knees position and felt so much groundedness and power in the intensity of each contraction.

I began to make sounds with each contraction as I rocked back and forth. The sounds were whale-like and were totally unconscious. I could feel them release the baby and open me. When a contraction subsided, I asked for a sip of tea or the tincture I had prepared for the birth.

During the labor I felt balanced and powerful unless someone

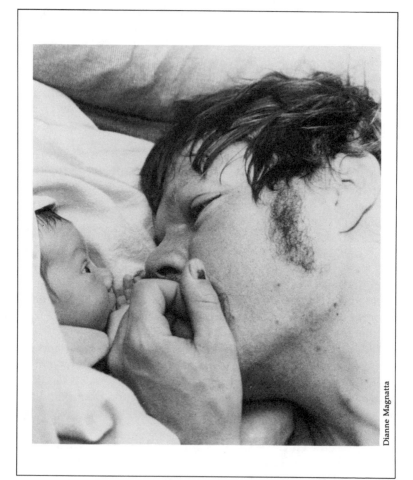

Dianne Magnatta

touched me. Then it was as if all my contained energy drained out through that person's touch, and I felt pain and lost my center.

When the baby's head crowned, I felt an intense ripping from my vagina to my clitoris which was very painful. Kathleen told me to pant. I said, "Fuck no!" and pushed with all my might. I couldn't imagine having that pain any longer. Pant? No, sorry. Push! And out he came.

In that instant there was complete silence. I held my breath. On my hands and knees I couldn't see him. All eyes and attention were on my new son. My thoughts in those seconds were: Oh, no,

I'm really a mother. How can I escape? Ahhh, it happened, it's over, take him away. Is he breathing? Is he whole? Does he have hair? Oh, Goddess, I hear him crying! Let me hold and love that sweet new one.

Then the room came to life. Yes, he was whole, bloody and beautiful. We had done it, he and I, and we were alive to enjoy it. A flood of relief surged through me and found release through tears. We did it in a powerful, sweet, intense two-hour labor.

Woman, Goddess, I thank you for the initiation into motherhood. Thank you, Grandmother, for showing me the strength, depth and mystery of life as female. Ignorance to knowledge, dark to light, never-ending circle. Atreyu Jaron was born on the first day of Hanukkah at sunset, the time of passage from dark to light, light to dark.

*Dianne grew up in Detroit and studied nursing before pursuing a career in the arts. She has received grants from the California Arts Council to establish an Art Center where she teaches pottery. Dianne says, "Jaron and I are partners in our large garden—he pulls up what I plant!"*

# My Quest

by Susan Root

---

Following the advice of a friend, I waited until I couldn't wait a moment longer before I made the decision to have a baby. That moment arrived on my thirtieth birthday and from then on I couldn't think of anything else; I was on a quest. Luckily I got pregnant almost immediately, but not before I read everything I could about infertility and regretted all those years of birth control pills, IUDs, creams, jellies, sponges and condoms. I identified with all women trying to have a baby, and I would, from then on, feel sympathetic to any woman's attempt to have a child.

Once I was pregnant, the course of my quest changed. My task was to find the situation that would provide the prenatal care and birth I envisioned. Unfortunately, my only two encounters with birth had given me a warped view of the process. The first birth that I witnessed was in a large county hospital where I worked. The birth was completely orchestrated by an intern and various other robed and masked figures—the woman on the delivery table seemed almost superfluous. Although I was awestruck by the phenomenon of birth, I also felt humiliated for all women who had their babies this way. The woman had just accomplished an amazing feat, had actually given birth to another human being, and no one seemed to be aware that she was even there. I was very young at the time, but I cried when I left the delivery room and knew I wouldn't *ever* let that happen to me.

The second birth I witnessed was a homebirth, in a foreign country, of a very close friend. I was to be her main support person, even delivering the baby should she be unable to locate anyone more qualified. My only qualifications were having witnessed one hospital birth and having read *Spiritual Midwifery*. Nevertheless, we were undaunted; we both felt capable and confident in her ability to birth normally and in mine to assist the natural process. We were *so* self-confident, in fact, that when a medical student offered to help, we accepted almost disdainfully. But I must admit that I will be forever grateful for his presence at the stillbirth of my friend's son. We shed tears together in sorrow for her dead baby, but the skill of the medical student saved my friend from additional physical suffering and saved me from a lifetime of guilt had I been there alone and incapable of helping her. My confidence in the birth process and in my own ability ever to have a live birth was severely shaken.

So, when my time came to make decisions involving my pregnancy and birth, neither the technically superior hospital birth nor the do-it-yourself homebirth seemed the right approach for me. I realized both were extremes and hoped that I could find a middle course. After ruling out an obstetrician, whose reply to my questions regarding the safety of homebirths was to compare it to giving birth in a cornfield, and the Clinic because the midwife program was in its earliest stages, I decided to have my baby at our small local hospital. Although the hospital had not yet embraced the "natural childbirth" philosophy, I felt that a newly employed young physician was likely to be persuaded to accommodate my wishes. He was, but at the time I was unaware of the influence of the larger powers within the institution; I was definitely going against the grain of how things were done. My doctor assured me that I would have the birth the way I wanted: no shave or enema; no episiotomy; Leboyer bath for the baby; my husband and friends in the delivery room (there was no birthing room at the time); no anesthesia or unnecessary medication; and rooming-in. He volunteered to come in for the birth, even if he wasn't on call. This was a real breach of hospital policy, I was told, but it did ensure my peace of mind and made me feel empowered.

When my labor began two weeks after my due date, I was very eager to get on with it; I had loved being pregnant, but I was definitely ready to exchange being a madonna to become a mother. When I felt the first contraction at four in the morning, my heart started racing with excitement. I restrained myself from waking my husband Ron right away; I lay back and enjoyed watching the clock, marveling at the rhythm of the contractions and the predictable intervals in between. I felt calm and very much in control when I woke Ron at 6:00 a.m.

It was my idea to remain at home as long as possible—I didn't want to get to the admitting room and be told I wasn't far enough along; nor did I want to be under the influence of the hospital any longer than necessary. But, at 8:00 a.m. when we were finally underway on the winding country road, I realized that we should have left before the contractions required so much of my attention. At that point I was no longer marveling at them; I was nauseous and torn between insisting that Ron stop the car so he could focus on me and help me breathe, and demanding that he drive faster . . . or slower, whichever seemed appropriate to me at the moment. I felt I had lost my grip on things and wished that I had been able to stay home. But I was grateful for those first two hours of labor

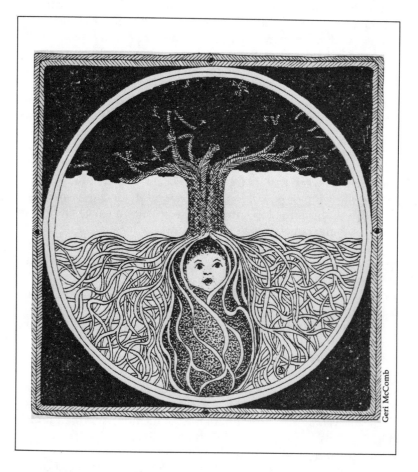

alone when I had felt so in tune; I *knew* that I was going to get through it.

When we arrived at the hospital, I literally ran down the hall to the labor room between contractions—I couldn't wait for a wheel-chair. The nurses followed with their prep kit, ready to give me the standard shave and enema. I frantically explained that if they'd just look on my chart, they would see the notation by my doctor that I didn't need to undergo their standard procedure. I breathed a sigh of relief when they removed their instruments. First battle won!

The labor was quick and predictable. I was only mildly irritated by the constant blood pressure and dilation checks. By noon I was on the delivery room table struggling to get the knack of pushing my baby out and feeling very ineffective flat on my back and with my feet in stirrups. My three closest friends were only allowed to watch from the doors of the delivery room, and I was too occupied to voice my dismay and change the situation. The nurse who was monitoring the baby's heartbeat added an element of panic to the birth by bringing in a senior staff physician who insisted that my doctor do an episiotomy to hurry things up because the baby's heart rate was dropping. After a small incision, my next push brought forth the baby's head, and the rest of the body seemed to slide right out.

The baby was given a very makeshift and unsatisfactory version of the Leboyer bath, and then we were whisked away, past my friends, to a room with "Isolation" posted on the door. The only way my doctor could arrange for rooming-in, which was against the hospital's policy, was to falsely state that I had a herpes infection, thereby preventing my baby from being in the nursery where he might contaminate the other infants. Although I technically got the rooming-in that I had wanted, the plan backfired because I was isolated from my friends, with whom I most wanted to share my joy. I felt very much alone that night and there was a time, about three o'clock in the morning, when I wished that I could have sent my crying baby to the nursery. I was exhausted; my adrenalin had finally worn off.

Essentially I had the birth that I wanted, but I felt that I had been deprived of some of its joy by not having the personal power to make it happen *exactly* as I wanted. I knew that the next time I became pregnant I would feel more confident in the ability of my body, and maybe I'd reconsider a homebirth. But I would have plenty of time to think about that later; right now I was too awestruck by the miracle of the birth of my son Teitan and too much in love with him to think of anything else. The *perfect* birth would have to be a future quest.

## THE TELEPHONE BABY

When the thought occured to me that pregnancy could be the cause of my nauseous stomach and missed period, I felt despondent and depressed; I hadn't planned this second pregnancy. Raising a lively two year old and helping to build our home seemed the limit of my ability and energy. I didn't have the time or desire to pursue a quest for a perfect birth. To make matters worse, I had an extremely nasty flu, and my body seemed to be a hostile environment for a newly developing fetus. I lay in bed feeling tearful, miserable and worried; I thought about miscarriages, abortions, sick babies and raising two children. As I sank into a mood of self-pity, I distinctly heard an inner voice say, *It's a healthy baby girl.* I thought, What? Did I just think that to make myself feel better? Then I heard it again, louder: *IT'S A HEALTHY BABY GIRL!* I couldn't ignore it that time—with those words my fear and misery were transformed into relief and joy. I went to sleep that night thinking about the daughter I had always wanted.

The next morning as I looked at the positive results of a home pregnancy test, I felt a rush of excitement—my intuition was confirmed and I was confident that I would have a healthy baby girl. But I knew that this pregnancy was going to be different. With my first I had focused on the birth as an end, a goal, an achievement; this time I thought of the pregnancy and birth only as a brief prelude to parenthood.

Having confidence in my ability to birth normally and hoping for a more empowering experience, I chose the Clinic for my prenatal care. I looked forward to my visits with Kate and Lorraine; it seemed like a time of emotional unburdening. I was able to confide in them the guilt I felt about my pragmatic attitude toward this pregnancy and birth and my fear that I was somehow cheating my second child by not having the same depth of awe and excitement that I'd had with my first. Lorraine and Kate reassured me that my feelings were normal and my guilt unnecessary; they helped me through the emotional rough spots of a normal pregnancy. I don't actually remember deciding to have a homebirth with the assistance of the midwives, but that decision was the outcome of the respect I felt for them and the confidence I had in their ability.

It was nearly the end of my pregnancy before I was forced to focus my full attention on it. I had been pleased about my relatively small size for being eight months pregnant but my prenatal exam

ended my feelings of satisfaction. Lorraine expressed concern because my uterine measurement was smaller than she would expect
for my dates and because it had not increased from the previous
week's measurement. She explained that the fundal height, measured in centimeters, usually coincides with the number of weeks'
gestation: at thirty-six weeks, mine was 30 centimeters.

I was totally unprepared for the discussion that followed among
Lorraine, Kate and Dr. Bill. Suddenly my perfectly "normal" pregnancy was being referred to in abnormal terms. Intrauterine fetal
growth retardation was the medical term for the condition that was
suspected. The consensus was that a sonogram would show if
there was a major problem causing the fetus to be undersized.

Since I'd had such a strong intuition that I was carrying a
healthy baby girl, I found it difficult to relate to their concern.
However, I perceived that I no longer had a choice, particularly if
I wanted the homebirth I had planned. I reluctantly arranged an
appointment with the radiologist for the next day.

I was totally preoccupied with thoughts of the sonogram and
wondered what to expect. How would my baby look? Would we
be able to determine its sex? What if it wasn't a girl? What if there
really was a serious problem? That night I had a vivid dream in
which I experienced a sonogram. Together with the doctor I examined the baby's vital parts: the brain, the spinal column, the heart.
Everything was normal and healthy. I awoke feeling calm, reassured and convinced that I was submitting to a needless procedure.

I was surprised at how similar my dream experience was to the
actual sonogram. Ron and I watched a squiggly mass of dots on a
screen—our baby. The doctor pointed out some of the identifiable
parts: the beating heart, a leg, a hand, the placenta. I asked if he
could tell the sex and he replied, "You don't want to know, do
you?" At that moment I didn't—the atmosphere wasn't right for
such a revelation. It would be another two days before we knew
the results of his measurements and calculations.

I could hardly restrain myself from calling Dr. Bill at the earliest
possible moment Monday morning. It was like a mini-birth experience hearing him say everything looked fine and normal with no
obvious physical defects, although the baby was indeed small.
From the measurement of the head, arm and leg bones, the
radiologist estimated the baby's weight to be less than four pounds.
The placenta was showing normal signs of deterioration which
were appropriate for my dates and confirmed that I was nearing

full term. I felt so relieved and elated when I hung up: I assumed that my premonition that all was well had been affirmed.

My high spirits were short-lived. At my next prenatal appointment I was unprepared for continued concern. The results of the sonogram did not dispel the anxiety as I had expected. My measurement that week was the same as the previous week. The recommendation was for a follow-up sonogram to measure the fetal growth over a two-week period. There was the possibility that the placenta was not functioning properly and not supplying the baby with enough nutrients to grow. A weak or insufficient placenta would not provide enough oxygen during labor contractions. Another concern was how a baby estimated to weigh less than four pounds would manage the stress of labor.

I began to realize that a homebirth was becoming an improbable idea as our discussion progressed to an explanation of stress tests administered at the hospital to see how the baby's heart would react to Pitocin-induced contractions. I felt very tearful and confused. My intuitive feeling that I had a strong, healthy, *little* baby girl was being undermined by hard medical facts. Statistics were clouding the clear picture I once had.

The second sonogram was uneventful without the intrigue of the first experience. The results would be ready in time for me to take them to the specialist in two days. The course seemed inevitable. I no longer felt I was a candidate for a homebirth. Although I was disappointed, I appreciated the caution with which the midwives worked. I did not want to become a statistic against the safety of homebirths. Despite my inner voice nagging me, *Everything is OK! It's a strong, healthy, little girl*, I resigned myself to the idea of a hospital birth. I no longer felt comfortable with the thought of a homebirth.

It was a week before my due date, but I had convinced myself and the midwives that this baby, like my first, would be two weeks late, giving it time to grow stronger and larger. I was experiencing abdominal cramping throughout the day, which I attributed to a relapse of an intestinal flu. There was no pattern to the cramps (it seemed an hour would go by between them), so I didn't pay much attention to my discomfort as I worked in the garden and prepared a big dinner for guests.

Following dinner, our friend Jim, who is an acupressurist, noticed my increasing discomfort and suggested a gentle massage. The massage was very soothing, but when he was done, my cramps worsened to the point that I could no longer enjoy conversing. I apologized and retired for the night.

When Ron came to bed at 12:45 a.m., I suggested that if he wanted a peaceful night's sleep, he should consider the couch. I explained that I had been getting up and down with bouts of cramps, vomiting and diarrhea. In fact, the cramps were getting so intense I was even trying some of the Lamaze breathing that I vaguely remembered from my first birth. I recall thinking that I really needed a refresher course before going into labor with this pregnancy.

After Ron watched me endure a couple of my cramps, which by this time were getting much stronger and more frequent, he said, "I'm concerned about these cramps! Are you sure they don't have anything to do with the baby? Maybe we should call one of the midwives." I was shocked. It hadn't even occurred to me that the baby was responsible for my discomfort. I even felt irritated by his impertinence.

I replied testily, "Of course it has nothing to do with the baby! I'm not calling anyone at one o'clock in the morning because I've got an intestinal flu!" The words were no sooner out of my mouth than I felt a strange popping sensation and a rush of warm water between my legs. Feeling very surprised and humble, I admitted that maybe he should try to call Kate or Lorraine.

After several calls, he finally reached Lorraine at the hospital where she was assisting with a long labor. It was 1:15 a.m., and Lorraine was calmly asking me how I was doing. I replied, on the verge of hysteria, "Awful! I already feel like pushing, I don't remember the breathing, and I don't have any idea what I'm doing!" She reassured me in a firm and composed voice that I was "doing it" and "doing it fine." Her voice had a miraculously calming effect on me. I explained that Ron was hastily gathering the birth pack I had prepared and putting my things into the car for the forty-minute drive to the hopital. She firmly instructed me not to leave the house; she would send an ambulance. She suggested that until it arrived, I lie on the bed and she would coach me through the contractions. Hearing her breathing on the other end was like a lifeline. Between contractions she gave an emergency childbirth class to Ron and Jim.

Despite all the panting and blowing I did, the baby was determined to emerge. I could feel the movement in the birth canal, and when I felt the stinging sensation, I knew that "blowing" wasn't going to stop anything. Ron was instructing me, "Blow! Blow! Don't push!" The look on his panic-stricken face framed by the "V" of my spread knees is still vivid. His eyes were so big and round with fear, I couldn't help but smile and try to sound reassuring as I informed him, "The baby is coming no matter what I do."

The head did the classic rotation as it came out. With the next contraction the shoulders and body seemed to tumble out. The loud cry immediately assured me that the baby was strong and healthy. Ron said, "Looks like we have a girl here." As he handed her to me, I felt such a rush of relief and disbelief. Less than an hour before, I had thought I had the flu.

The ambulance attendants arrived in time to congratulate us and clamp the cord. They offered us a ride back to the hospital, which we declined. Although the baby looked small, she was very alert, and her heartbeat, pulse and respiration were satisfactory.

The next day Lorraine came to make sure we were all doing well. Her examination of the baby indicated that she was full term and weighed four pounds, eight ounces. The placenta was very small with a portion of it flattened and tough, which supported the suspicion of placental insufficiency.

My intuitive feelings were put through a test by Alexis' birth, but they proved to be right. But so, too, were the technological speculations. The only explanation I can give for being unaware at the beginning stages of labor is that it wasn't at all like my first labor and that I wasn't meant to know. If the thought of the impending birth had emerged into my conscious mind, I would have felt compelled to seek specialized medical care; that just wasn't meant to be. While medical facts, calculations and statistics definitely have their place in the evaluation of a particular situation, a pregnant woman's intuition rates an added measure of confidence and credibility. There is a very unique and special bond between a mother and her unborn child.

*Before having children, Susan and Ron lived and traveled extensively in foreign countries. Susan dreams of satisfying her wanderlust by combining her children's education with life in a foreign culture. In the meantime, she and Ron continue work on their solar home, manage their eighty acre homestead and raise organic apples and pears.*

# For Michael

by Gail Eastwood

---

The day you were born was such a rich and deep time that I could write dozens of stories about it—each one different, and each one true. Here's one true story:

Christmas Day! It was a dandy day for a party, and everyone was here "on the land," including my parents and my two brothers. But even before noon, as we were getting ready for Christmas dinner, it became clear from the regularity of my contractions that a different party was going to happen. I was amazed at the way my abdomen would mound up so tightly of its own bidding. I was excited as we timed the contractions and called Lorraine, our midwife, on the CB radio.

As evening neared, I was hurting more with the contractions and was in the bathtub trying to relax. My friend Mu'frida stayed to sit with us for the night, "holding the light." I thought I could handle the pain at that point but was getting anxious for the midwives to appear.

They came at last in the evening, having barely finished the plum pudding at their Christmas dinner. Lorraine examined me—I was only a centimeter dilated, no more than I had been two weeks before. She asked, "Could you sleep?"

I was crushed knowing there was no way I could sleep in so much pain, and doubting I could handle the long slow labor she was anticipating. Mu'frida, watching, reached me with the instruction to stop judging: "Be gentle with yourself."

Lorraine suggested an enema. She said it would either speed or slow the labor. And, indeed, it did seem to lend more force to the contractions which had been lagging since Lorraine and Becca's arrival. Becca went to bed, having been up all of Christmas Eve at another birth, and Lorraine prepared to stay up with us.

I wonder what you were experiencing: sounds, movements, energies—much like those of the preceding months. And yet different—energies changing one another, gathering, harmonizing, potentizing. Did the profound change frighten, disturb, excite you? You were not then so separate from us—or from the universe—as you would later learn to be. We were all working together

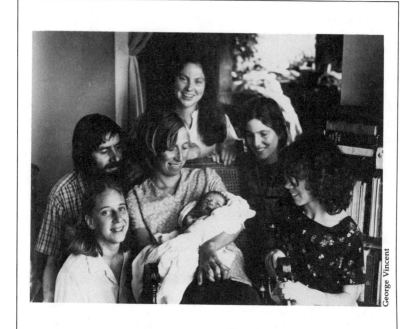

George Vincent

in this event, disregarding our little separate selves as best we could. I was working with you, of course, but I was not listening to you much that night. Later I could only guess at your state of mind. I think you were mainly watchful, like Bill, your father, who sat on his meditation pillow all night, holding me with his eyes.

And me—I was watching and listening to pain, to my own breathing, sustained by my awareness of those around me. My memory of the passing of the night is not sequential. I remember having no tolerance for odors or even for touching. Poor Bill could not squeeze in a sandwich or a caress. There was pain. If I thought of continuing all night, I would feel discouraged; if I stayed with the present pain, each contraction was manageable, each moment was possible. The only other thing that I had room for in my consciousness was the supporting awareness of our "team"—those with us in flesh and blood, and many others besides. I asked Lorraine to examine me—4 centimeters. We were progressing.

As the pain increased I wanted to tense and rise up out of it. Mu'frida kept reminding me to send my breath all the way down, to sink into the contraction, to feel my connection with the ground. Joan, another friend, plied me with Rescue Remedy, a Bach flower essence, and I think she plied the others with tea. I breathed out slowly to Bill, "hu," which meant to me, "love, only love."

I had tried a number of positions—curled on my side, on my knees, sitting propped on pillows. Lorraine suggested I stand. What an outrageously impossible idea! But I had no choice except to try anything that might help. I "stood" with Bill supporting me, carrying the weight as each contraction took over. Sure enough, my waters broke and things intensified.

Now the team went into faster action. Becca was awakened, tools were gathered. An exam showed my dilation well progressed. It was hard not to push. "Pant," said Lorraine.

At last it was time to push. Lorraine was a good teacher as always. She gave me one good pointer at a time, watched to see how I worked with it, then gave me the next piece of information I needed. "Make a low sound" she prompted, demonstrating, "oooh," in a deep low voice.

I'm not sure I had really been saying "eek," in a tight high voice before, but that's how I felt. "Oooh," I attempted. My team clustered around in front of me with wide open eyes and mouths. "Oooh," they chorused, deep and intense. "Oooh," I replied, playacting the sound, deep and commanding until it took over. I was sounding and pushing with all the energy that was available, myself a part, but only a part, of the action.

They told me of your head advancing and retreating. "Feel it," said Becca between contractions. It was hard and warm. Finally your head was out. You were sucking furiously at the syringe as they tried to suction out the mucus. I was reclining, perched above the floor on a pillow.

"Do you want to catch the baby?" Lorraine asked Bill. The rest of the pushing wasn't hard, and anyway I was too much in shock from the power of that transition to notice. Your father was the first to hold you. Soon your small body lay on top of mine. You were crying, I think. What were you aware of? I was lost, but soon you were loudly (and not for the last time) calling me to myself.

Your father held you on his bare chest. The placenta came out easily while I was still in a fog. You were becoming more and more unhappy, your breathing disturbed, and Lorraine was preparing to take you to the emergency room. Everybody gave you what they could. What worked? Your cries subsided, you took the breast. As the soft December light dawned, your eyes, tightly closed at first, opened wide, gazing raptly at the light.

A photograph taken that morning shows you looking seriously at the world with those so-wide eyes, us looking at you. You drinking in the light of the world, us drinking in the light of you. I was confused and changed, shaken, didn't know myself. I look a bit tentative in the picture. Bill's face is soft, gentle, a shy radiance opening. You seem watchful and in command of the situation.

The house where you were born was built with the dream of you in my mind, the power of that dream backing every nail I drove. But what dream could hold a candle to the fleshly reality of a dream come true?

I'll tell you this story and perhaps others about the same event when you get a little older. Wouldn't I love, though, to hear yours!

*Gail built her own home before falling in love with Bill. For the past nine years they have been building ferro-cement water tanks for a livelihood. They grow all of their vegetables and fruits organically and keep goats, which supply them with a bounty of milk and cheese. Gail, who has a masters degree in clinical social work from the University of California at Berkeley, has a lifelong interest in how people effect change in their lives. She has studied biokinesiology for seven years and currently has a part-time private practice.*

# A Matter
# of the Heart

by Marie Mintz

It is with great hesitation that I sit down to write this birth story, because I know it will dredge up some very unpleasant memories for me. The time of Simone's birth, six years ago, was the most intensely emotional period of my life. I felt totally ecstatic, exhilarated and filled with love; yet the weeks following her birth were the most painful I'd ever experienced.

The labor and delivery were quick, only four hours. I was so elated to have had an easy birthing at home during the quiet of the early dawn. It was, to my mind, just perfect—a beautiful, intimate experience shared by those closest to me.

However, Simone, our first child, was born with a birth defect. She had a strange lump the size of a large marble on the top of her head. Although she seemed otherwise healthy, there was no ignoring the lump. Kate, our midwife, had never seen anything like it, and it worried her enough to send us to the hospital right away. From then on the elation and joy we felt at the birth were coupled with a nightmarish series of x-rays, CAT scans, specialists, and a lot of poking and probing of the baby whom we had so tried to give a tranquil start in life.

The first few doctors we saw didn't know quite what to make of the lump. They were trying to determine if it contained any brain matter. One doctor invited me to sit in his office when he saw me pacing and sobbing outside the x-ray room where Simone was screaming. (Eddie and I took turns holding her during those procedures.) The doctor proceeded to tell me that if a baby has one defect, chances are more will show up, and we should be prepared to raise a retarded child. Devastating as this information was, it didn't matter. The love we felt for our child was so strong that we didn't care what was wrong with her. I felt like I had just joined humanity. I understood all mothers everywhere and their unceasing devotion to their children. The old expression, "Only a mother could love," made so much more sense to me. Always before, in matters of the heart, I had been cautious. It was a new experience for me to be so totally and instantly in love, and hence rendered so vulnerable. It was a very scary feeling.

Another overwhelming new feeling was that of having total responsibility for another human being. This feeling was made all the more intense in the face of the constant medical decisions we were confronted with. We felt powerless against the medical establishment, thinking that if we didn't agree to various suggested procedures it would be endangering Simone's life.

One such test involved sticking a tube into a vein in Simone's thigh that led to her brain and then injecting dye through the tube into her brain to illuminate the blood vessels in her head—at ten days old! The whole procedure sounded ghastly, and my instant reaction was, "No way! How can you possibly stick a tube into the vein of a newborn baby?" After many reassurances ("We do it all the time") and the implication that it was a necessary preoperative procedure, we reluctantly agreed to it. The doctors and medical students ended up poking at Simone's leg for two and a half hours while she was anesthetized and failed to get the tube into her vein. I was furious at them but more at myself—I should have stuck to my intuition and refused to allow them to do it in the first place. As it turned out, the procedure wasn't absolutely necessary, and they could operate anyway. They said the test "would have been like a roadmap, but we can just stop for directions along the way." Why hadn't they told us that before? Oh, to have known then what I know now.

It had been determined by a CAT scan that the lump on Simone's head did not contain brain matter. Now the problem was removing it without doing any damage to the brain. When she was thirteen days old, they operated. At that point I was a physical and emotional wreck—recovering from the birth, getting used to nursing and sleeping in a rocking chair next to Simone's little isolette. Luckily I had lots of help from wonderful friends, and Eddie was right there when I crumpled from it all. The surgery was a success, the lump was removed, and finally we were able to leave the hospital, Simone with a shaved and bandaged head.

For about two years I allowed for the possibility that Simone might be retarded, even though the doctors assured me she wasn't. If another child her age said "Mommy" before she did, I would wonder. After a few years, it became clear that she was normal. We were lucky, but it gave me an idea of what it would be like to deal with a handicapped child—you just do it.

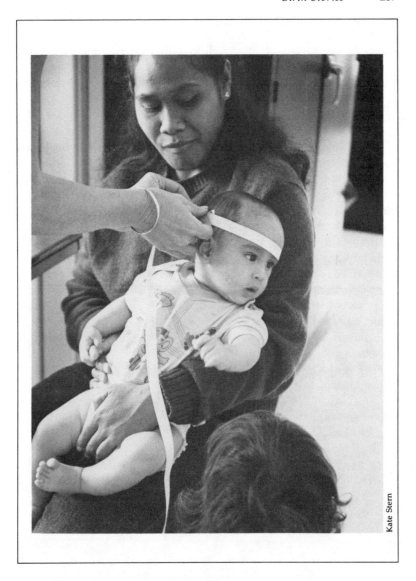

Kate Stern

We went to genetic counselors to find out what we could, but they really couldn't give us any reasons for the lump. When I became pregnant with my second child, I had a sense of uneasiness. I felt that we'd gotten off easy the first time and that this baby might have some major defects. I decided to have amniocentesis as the odds of having a second child with a neural tube defect are greater. (Neural tube defects occur about 1 in every thousand births. Once a couple has had a child with such a defect, the chance of recurrence is 2 per hundred.)

At that point I was very confused about what I would do if the baby turned out to have something wrong with it. After all, Simone's amniotic fluid might have indicated a defect, and yet it turned out to be relatively minor. Would I have aborted her if I had known?

The whole realm of amniocentesis is full of complex questions, and I wonder, is it better to know these things? And then, how do you act upon the knowledge? Amniocentesis is done in the fourth month of pregnancy, and it takes approximately three weeks to get the results. This waiting period was a very difficult time. I went over and over in my mind, What will I do if . . . ? I've known of children with Down's syndrome who have enriched the lives of their families immeasurably. To have an abortion in the fourth or fifth month is a much more complex procedure than if done earlier. I felt very removed from my pregnancy at a time when I should have been enthusiastically embracing it. I was, however, greatly relieved to find out that my baby was fine, but I did carry a residual tension throughout the pregnancy from those early months of uncertainty.

Lorraine, Kate, Kathleen and Alison were at my second homebirth. They massaged me throughout my labor (delightful! How can you do anything but relax when four sets of hands are rubbing you?), and there was Jasper. We all held our breath as the midwives checked him—perfect. How amazing!

*Marie and her family have moved to the San Francisco Bay Area so that she can continue her education. She plans to combine genetic counseling with social work in order to help parents with situations similar to hers.*

# Garth's Journey

by Kathy Epling

It is nearly six years now since I first met Lorraine. She won my heart by the simple and perfect way she said, "Hello, baby," while feeling my yet-to-be-born child's position and size beneath my rounded, stretched skin. "Have you thought about what kind of birth you want?" she asked.

I shrugged and said, "Well, a safe and easy one at home." I didn't want friends there, except John, the baby's father, or any of the trappings of the more imaginatively romantic settings I'd read of. But I definitely wanted my November child—due, I was certain, precisely on November 25, Saint Catherine's Day, day of a full moon—to be born with ease and love at home.

I spent my pregnant months reading birth stories and looking in awe at women with new babies: They had done it, they had been there, they were walking around holding their little babies as if nothing had happened.

And then, October 25, night of a full moon, night of a storm, I started feeling some strange tightenings in my back and belly. Not labor, certainly. But then, what were they? Unusually strong Braxton-Hicks contractions? John and I drove out to Lorraine's home (a good practice drive, I figured, for the day he'd have to find it quickly). Or, we tried to drive there. We wandered lost through horse meadows under the full moon, laughing at how crazy it was, and thought, No, this isn't labor, couldn't be. Finally a kind soul passing by gave us clear directions, and we made it to Lorraine's little home which was all lit up, music coming from the radio inside. Hooray!

But she wasn't there. A friend who was staying with Lorraine's son Devlin said she was out of town and might not be back that night since there was a storm due. "Oh well," I said (this wasn't labor after all, it would go away soon). And I left her a note.

In town, belying my apparent calm, I went to every possible place she might go, laying a trail of notes ("It's really all right, but I'd like to see you . . . "): at the Clinic, a friend's house, the movie theatre. We stopped at the liquor store for ice cubes (this wasn't labor, but it might be good to have ice to suck if . . . ), and then went to our bookstore for a copy of *Emergency Childbirth*. I stayed up all night reading portions of it to John. (Not that it was labor, of course, but why not be ready for anything?)

At work in the bookstore the next day, the strange tightenings were not going away, but neither were they very troublesome. I got out the obstetric texts and peered at drawings of cervixes dilating, babies emerging. I phoned the Clinic—"No, Lorraine isn't in, she works next Tuesday." It was Thursday, the twenty-sixth. I went home on my lunch break and cried. I knew if necessary I could give birth alone, but I was suddenly feeling mighty lonely.

Later that afternoon I opened my door and there was Lorraine. It felt like a visitation from an angel or the arrival of the cavalry: All would be well. She examined me and said I was totally effaced and, yes, I was having contractions. She told me I should get the birth supplies ready and contact her when things intensified. Her assistant, Jody, would be staying in town, and she could stay with me when John went to get Lorraine.

Mad exhilaration. Shopping on Friday: white shoelaces, rubbing alcohol, sanitary towels. Bubbling over to the woman at the pharmacy: "My baby is coming! I need to buy these things."

She was so kind and supportive. "Yes, lots of babies get born at home these days. Good luck!" And working at the bookstore, I had to stop talking during contractions, but they were still gentle.

Early Saturday morning the mucus plug came out and things felt more intense. "This is it," I told John. "Send Jody here and get Lorraine." It was about 3:00 a.m., October 29.

Jody arrived, full of gentle excitement. I had not met her before, but liked her. "Your baby's coming!" she said. I felt like dancing with excitement, yet I also felt a certain disbelief: A baby? Really?

John and Lorraine got back quickly, and we settled in—water boiling on the stove, conversation, support. I was having back labor, and it felt good to have John press his hand firmly on the small of my back during contractions. Such amazing power, those surges through my body. I tried to watch them, examine them: There is pressure here, spreading, a sense of heat, of opening. Now it is going, and finally—stillness. The space between contractions surprised me, so clear, so lovely. Time to gather energy once again.

I was dilating slowly, so to speed and strengthen the contractions I tried dancing—bends, lunges, turns. They felt good. I felt strong, supported by the three people with me. As I breathed through contractions, Lorraine reminded me to keep my muscles relaxed and to open my eyes. (I was closing them and getting lost in the pain, overwhelmed. With my eyes open to the ordinary things of the now sunlit room, it was easier.) Ice and honey, valerian tea, legs shaking, vomiting. Soon, soon, soon.

Midafternoon Saturday. The contractions had slowed, eased. I felt very calm, very slow. The sunlight made rainbows on the walls as Devlin spun a prism in my window. Everyone left me alone for a time. Lorraine stayed outside on the porch within the sound of my voice should I call. I sat calmly and sang to my child and to myself, and watched the birds in the garden and thought about the child, about mothering.

My support people came back, and we went through another night. They took turns sleeping, but I didn't sleep—I had no need to, floating as I was on their loving energy. Intense contractions, yet still I was dilating so slowly. More standing, stretching, dancing. How I longed to take control, but I couldn't even feel my cervix opening. I tried to imagine a morning glory unfolding, opening, releasing my child. Always Lorraine, Jody or John was there, touching me, telling me I was strong, holding me.

Long night. I knew Jody was worried; Lorraine seemed untroubled. I felt all was well. But it was going on so long. Daylight came again; it was Sunday, October 30. More hours of storm and sunlight, more contractions and more and more. And still those loving people beside me, lifelines holding me to this world, pulling me through the long journey.

At 5:00 p.m., Lorraine phoned the doctor who had examined me, and he advised that I go to the hospital. We sat in a circle, the four of us. Lorraine said she'd stay with me as long as I wished to go on. I asked what was likely to happen at the hospital and what was slowing the labor. And we talked and talked. I tried a hot bath and the contractions intensified but dilation did not speed up. I looked at the tired faces of those loving people, thought of my child, thought of the easy, safe homebirth I'd hoped for, and said, "OK, I'll go to the hospital."

Lorraine couldn't come with John and me—those were the days of uneasy relations between the midwives and the hospital. So we went alone and said we had intended to birth at home, but it had gone on so long we decided to come in. I held John's hand and said, "He's staying with me. And I don't want any drugs, and please give me my baby as soon as it's born, and can you dim the lights?" I had a fierce determination to control the situation as much as I could. The people at the hospital were fairly good about it.

The doctor broke the bag of water and three times offered me Demerol to "take the edge off," and three times I smiled and said, "No, I'm fine, thank you."

The nurse, when I said I was feeling a strong urge to push, said, "Don't, you've got hours yet to go." So I tried not to push, but it was hard. And then, while sloshing disinfectant over my thighs, she exclaimed, "My God, that's your baby's head!" and ran for the doctor.

I smiled at John and said, "Well, catch it if it comes out now." But the doctor and the nurses returned and quickly moved me to the delivery room. ("No, I will not lie down. I feel more comfortable sitting up a little.") Pushes and pushes and pushes. I watched in the big round mirror—could that be my baby's head coming out, going back and coming out? Push! Push! And then the head was out, and the shoulders, and the body. The baby was placed on my belly as I was still peering into the mirror, dazed and happy, watching my rose-colored child cry.

"Look at your son," said the nurse. I did, and I reached down to touch him and felt such pity and love. I held him and nursed him, and would not release him to the nursery—having waited so long I would not let him go now. Wide eyes, strange but known face. "Garth," I said. "Garth, where did you really come from?"

We went home to the house that Jody and Lorraine had cleaned for me while I had been at the hospital, and we slept.

So that was Garth's birth. The next day Lorraine returned to greet the baby she had helped bring forth and to answer my questions. That was the beginning of my birth into motherhood. But that's another story, still going on.

## HOME FREE

Garth was nearly seven years old the summer he and I stared at the floating dark ring in a home pregnancy test and I said, "It means a baby."

It had been seven years of changes. When Garth was three, his father and I ended our romantic-sexual relationship, though we remained friends and business associates. When Garth was five, we moved to share our lives with my longtime friend and love, Paul, in his small hand-built cabin, forty minutes from town.

The previous winter, I had had an early miscarriage, so early very few people knew of it; but the grief I carried tinged all the days of spring. This new pregnancy bore the weight of many expectations and fears. Although Paul loved Garth, he had never wanted to be a biological father, and the prospect of fatherhood at forty-seven awed him. At thirty-seven I felt it was a last-chance child, a great blessing. One July afternoon soon after the positive test I stood a while in my garden looking into the open cup of a white lily, shaken with joy and fear. Would this child stay? What would the birth bring? "Grow safe, grow strong," I told my child, who by then would have fit on the tip of a match.

"The heart is beating!" I announced one day after studying a fetal growth chart.

Paul looked at me in astonishment. "Can you feel it?"

"No, no, I won't feel the child for months yet. But the heart starts now."

I contacted Lorraine early in the pregnancy. I remember the relief, the well-being that flooded through me the day she came into the bookstore where I work, hugged me, and we started talking of the coming child.

The child was due March 24. I felt it might come later, around the April full moon, on the fifth, but having been three weeks off with Garth's date, I made no firm pronouncements.

Months passed and the baby grew and kicked. Garth and Paul listened to the hummingbird-fast heartbeat. In the last weeks Paul began earnestly and nervously reading *Emergency Childbirth* every night. He went over and over the procedures and possibilities, and inexplicably found himself studying the maneuver to free stuck shoulders. I told him not to worry, that it was very unlikely.

I was busy at the bookstore and obsessed with readying my garden for the spring and summer. I planted old-fashioned rose bushes, blooming primroses and bulbs—bought with money sent to me for baby clothes. Meanwhile, the waterline broke, the chimney pipe on our woodstove collapsed, we ran out of firewood, and it snowed. I scrubbed the wooden floor of our untidy cabin and wondered if it—and we—would ever be ready for the birth.

The due date passed. The stovepipe and waterline were fixed; the snow melted. The forget-me-nots came into clear blue bloom, and the baby plum trees flowered. The moon neared full. Examining my cervix I found I could touch my baby's hard head. Lorraine said I was about 1½ centimeters dilated and partially effaced, but I was having no contractions.

Then, April 2, they began. Anticipating another long latent phase, I decided to go into town and pick up groceries, clear up final work at the bookstore (I had arranged to take three weeks off before returning to work with the baby) and see Lorraine. Unable to locate her at the Clinic, Garth, Paul and I walked to her yoga class, but she wasn't there. Would we find her? Her son Devlin whizzed by on his bike. "Hey, Kathy, are you in labor?"

"Yes!" I answered.

"Well, my mom is at Deborah's, but she'll be back soon." He promised to have her come see me at John's apartment above the bookstore.

As we waited, my mucus plug came out, copious and blood-streaked. Contractions were still fairly far apart and didn't last long, but I could no longer talk through them. I longed to be home.

When Lorraine came and checked me, she said I was at 4 centimeters, as was Deborah, whom she'd just checked. I laughed and said, "Deborah is first, I told her she could be." Lorraine said she'd see us that night for the baby's birth. Armed with phone numbers, juice and a new batch of baby plants for my garden, we headed home.

It was about four in the afternoon when we reached the cabin. While Paul and Garth tried to put things in order inside, I stayed in the garden tucking the little plants in: maiden pinks, veronica, snow in summer, columbines. It was good to feel the warmth of the April sunlight, good to be alone for a time.

I was feeling the contractions in my back as well as my belly, and they were fierce and strong. Good, I thought. Power. Let it open me up.

I went upstairs into our small sleeping room. Soon after, I asked Paul and Garth to stay with me. It helped the back pain if Paul pressed hard at the base of my spine, slightly to the right. I breathed through the waves of pressure and pain, and tried to relax.

About sunset, during a particularly hard contraction, our neighbor, Paul's sister Elaine, dropped by. She was worried—why wasn't the midwife here? I lost track of my breathing, cried out and called down to Paul, "Please, tell her to go home! Come upstairs! Tell her I'm fine, but please tell her to leave."

Elaine called up to me, "You sound pretty far along. Are you sure you're OK?"

The contraction over, I laughed, apologized for my rudeness and said, "I take days and days to birth my children. Everything is fine. We'll let you know when the baby comes." Not wholly reassured, she left.

But now the question was out in the open. When *were* we going to phone Lorraine? Paul would have to be gone nearly an hour while Garth, the coming child and I waited in the cabin. The contractions were seven minutes apart, then four minutes, then fifteen minutes, then ten minutes. There seemed no pattern to them, but they felt harder and harder. At about 7:30 p.m., I told Paul to try to reach Lorraine. Garth stayed with me, pressing with both hands against my back, very serious and still.

Paul returned with word that Lorraine was at Deborah's but would be leaving soon as Kate was also there.

Strong contractions. My whole body was shaking with their force. At 9:30 p.m., Lorraine and Alison came quietly into our candlelit home. Deborah, they said, had given birth to a big, dark-haired boy. I smiled at this news; Deborah *had* been first and all was well. Examining me, Lorraine said I was about 8 centimeters dilated—sweet words. My cervix was opening, my body was responding, these hard contractions had purpose. Ah, but they hurt amazingly. Walking outside, under a ripening moon, I clung to Lorraine through a couple of hard ones. I remember her soft, fragrant hair against my cheek. How reassuring it was to hold onto her for a moment.

Inside again. Alison and Garth dozed a little. One of our semi-tame skunks came darting through the loft. I was glad and amused to see her.

After a couple of hours Lorraine said I was fully open. But I felt no urge to push. When I pushed the pain intensified. "It hurts to push," I said.

Lorraine replied, "You'll have to push through the pain and come out on the other side." So I pushed. I pushed standing, holding on to Paul for dear life. I pushed squatting, hanging from his shoulders. How his back must ache, I thought. His face was drenched with sweat. I pushed again and again.

The baby would not clear my pelvic bones. I thought fleetingly of cesareans. Oh, please, no. How I wanted this homebirth. Push! Again! Push! "Baby," I said, "baby, we love you. We want to see

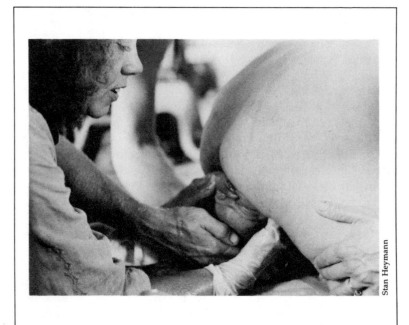

Stan Heymann

you. All you have to do is slide down. Just slide down. Easy. Now!"

Another contraction. Yes! The baby was moving down. Lorraine reached in to help reposition the baby's head so it would come through more directly.

I pushed for four hours and thought, Now I understand the meaning of the word *labor!* Alison suggested that I make noises while I pushed. What noises I made; even as I made them I wondered at them. They were deep, loud, huge, primal sounds. They reminded me of volcanoes and storms and herds of elephants. And they did help.

I leaned on our sleeping mats, Alison propping me up from behind—my sharp elbows probably left bruises on her arms for weeks. Lorraine knelt in front of me, a center of calm. Paul and Garth sat beside me quietly.

The head! Yes, the baby was coming! Yes! And now, not to push. Panting, blowing, stretching. Open, open, so open. Lorraine put my hand on the crowning, slippery baby head—amazement.

The head was out, the cord wrapped tightly around the neck

twice. The head turned and Lorraine deftly unlooped the cord, then said, "Push!"

"I'm not having a contraction," I objected.

"PUSH NOW!" she insisted. I pushed twice with no contractions while Lorraine freed my baby's stuck shoulders, and suddenly the baby slid out and was placed on my stomach. Lorraine and Alison massaged her. I stroked her gently, and she turned pink, began to breathe and cried a little—and then she was in my arms.

I laughed and cried and asked, "Oh, will she stay?"

"She's not going anywhere," smiled Lorraine.

Garth danced all over the room exclaiming, "This is more exciting than the landslide!" And Paul beamed.

"Laurel," I said, looking at my baby's dear face. My lovely girl, I thought, I have known you always. Welcome home, my darling.

Somewhere the placenta was being delivered. Someone was making tea. Alison called my name, asked if I was OK. Was I in shock?

I was fine, I told her with a smile, and went back to gazing at Laurel's face. She was safe, we were safe. "Home free," I whispered to her, "home free."

*Kathy works at a bookstore and manages a mailorder book business which specializes in children's books and books on pregnancy, birth and parenting. She is a poet and her poems have been widely published in literary magazines. With Paul, she publishes* The Peacemaker, *a monthly newsletter. She says, "My flowers are doing very well, and I would like to keep chickens someday, although I think doves would be prettier."*

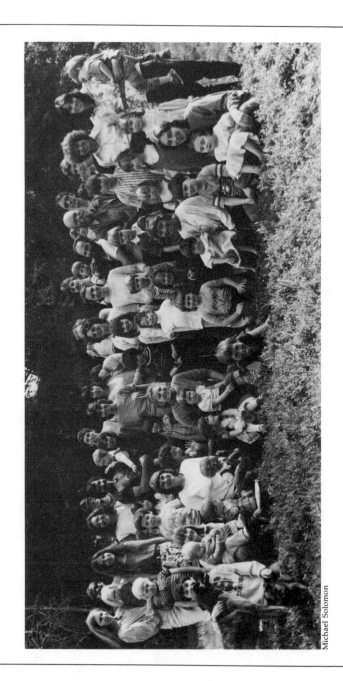

Michael Solomon

# Conclusion

For many women, giving birth is a miraculous event, a time of tremendous growth and change. Yet for our mothers and grandmothers, birth was kept a mystery by medical men who sought to control it; the hospital maternity ward was accepted as the safe and modern place to have babies. Later generations, however, found the routinely used manipulations and interventions dehumanizing and unpleasant, alienating them from an important experience in their lives. Today, women are reclaiming their birthing rights, and it is our hope that in sharing their birth stories, women will further understand the process and their individual power to take control.

Most of the birth stories in this collection would have gone unwritten without the inspiration of this book; recording the details of birth has not been a practice of our society. If you have ever asked your parents about the circumstances surrounding your own entry into this world, only to receive a very sketchy impression, then perhaps you know the value of creating a written account of one of the most significant occasions in your life—the bringing forth of a new life.

Composing a birth story does not require any special skills; few of the authors of these stories consider themselves to be writers. Once you overcome the obstacle of finding the time to collect your thoughts, all that is necessary is putting the facts and emotions that are important to you on paper. We have found that using a letter format, imagining that your child will read the story in later years, inspires ideas and helps you focus on what you want your child to know about the birth. We also suggest that the story be written as soon after the birth as possible while the memory is still fresh and clear; you will then be better able to write about the impact that the birth has had on your body and spirit.

It has been with pleasure and a sense of gratitude that we have shared these birth tales with you. We hope that you have gained a feeling of empowerment from them and that your pregnancy and birth experiences will be enriched. We are enthusiastic that this book will sow the seeds for a new tradition, a custom of sharing with our children the joy and magic of their beginnings.

# Glossary

**Amniocentesis:** A test of the amniotic fluid used to diagnose congenital and genetic defects of the fetus.

**Apgar score:** A test developed by Dr. Virginia Apgar to evaluate a newborn's condition, taken one minute after birth and again at five minutes.

**Asepsis:** Sterile; free from germs.

**Bach flower essence:** Wildflower extracts developed by Dr. Edward Bach used for natural healing.

**Back labor:** A labor in which the contractions are felt mainly in the lower back, occuring most frequently when the baby is in a posterior or breech position.

**Bilirubin lights:** Fluorescent lights used in the treatment of jaundice of the newborn.

**Bloody show:** The blood-tinged mucus plug that is discharged from the cervix at the onset of dilation.

**Bonding:** The forming of strong emotional attachments between a baby and its parents.

**Bradley method:** A method of birth preparation (called Husband-Coached Childbirth) developed by Dr. Robert Bradley, which uses relaxation techniques to control pain during labor.

**Braxton-Hicks contractions:** Mild, irregular contractions which strengthen the uterus before the onset of labor.

**Breech:** A position in which the baby's bottom, rather than its head, is the presenting part.

**Caput:** A medical term for the head.

**Castor oil:** A home remedy sometimes used to induce or stimulate labor.

**Caul:** A term for the amniotic sac.

**Cephalo-pelvic disproportion:** A condition in which the baby's head is too large to pass through the mother's pelvis, making a vaginal delivery impossible.

**Cervical lip:** A small portion of the cervix that has not receded, preventing complete dilation.

**Colostrum:** A protein-rich yellow fluid that precedes the breast milk and contains the mother's antibodies.

**Crowning:** When the crown of the baby's head is coming through the vaginal opening.

**Demerol:** A commonly used narcotic analgesic that works as a muscle relaxant to alleviate pain in the first stage of labor.

**Doula:** A woman trained to assist the mother during the perinatal period. The term and concept, also called "mothering the mother," were first described by Dana Raphael in *The Tender Gift: Breastfeeding*.

**Effacement:** The thinning of the cervix prior to and during the early stages of dilation.

**Engagement:** When the presenting part of the fetus, usually the head, has settled deep into the mother's pelvis.

**Epidural:** An anesthesia administered by a small catheter inserted in the epidural space surrounding the spinal cord to block sensation.

**Episiotomy:** A surgical incision in the perineum to enlarge the vaginal opening.

**External version:** The manual turning of the fetus to a presentation that facilitates delivery.

**Forewaters:** Amniotic fluid preceding the baby's head.

**Jin Shin Jyutsu treatments:** An ancient Japanese method of healing that uses techniques similar to acupressure to harmonize energy flows.

**Lact-Aid:** A device which enables an infant to receive formula through a small tube while suckling at the breast, stimulating lactation and providing the closeness of nursing for adoptive mothers. Manufactured by Lact-Aid, P.O. Box 1066, Athens, Tennessee 37303.

**Lamaze method:** A method of birth preparation developed by Dr. Fernand Lamaze which uses breathing techniques and relaxation to control pain during labor.

**Leboyer bath:** A technique developed by Dr. Frédérick Leboyer to reduce the trauma of birth by placing the newborn in warm water.

**Meconium:** A greenish-black tarry substance that is contained in the fetus' intestines.

**Mucus plug:** A substance in the cervix that seals the uterus from the vaginal canal during pregnancy.

**Nisentil:** A narcotic analgesic used to relieve pain during labor which relaxes the mother and has less of a depressant effect on the fetus than Demerol.

**Non-stress test:** Monitoring of the fetal heart rate, without the use of Pitocin to stimulate contractions, to evaluate the condition of the fetus.

**Occult umbilical prolapse:** Undetected prolapse cord.

**Palpate:** To examine by touch.

**Pelvic inflammatory disease:** Any of a group of infections of the female reproductive organs, which can lead to infertility.

**Perineum:** The area between the anus and the vagina that is often massaged to prevent tearing or the need for an episiotomy.

**Pitocin:** a synthetic hormone used to stimulate uterine contractions.

**Placenta abruptio:** Complete or partial separation of the placenta from the wall of the uterus, life-threatening to the mother and baby.

**Polyhydromnios:** Excessive amniotic fluid sometimes associated with diabetes, twins, toxemia and congenital malformations of the fetus.

**Posterior:** A presentation in which the back of the baby's head faces the mother's back.

**Prolapsed cord:** A condition in which the umbilical cord precedes the fetus into the birth canal, cutting off the oxygen supply if the cord is compressed.

**Shoulder dystocia:** An uncommon complication in which the baby's shoulders cannot be born without assistance.

**Sonogram:** A diagnostic test which produces a picture of the fetus through the use of high-frequency sound waves.

**Stages of labor:**
First: Dilation of the cervix.
Second: Expulsion of the baby.
Third: Expulsion of the placenta.

**Stress test:** Monitoring of the fetal heart rate, using Pitocin to stimulate contractions, to evaluate the condition of the fetus.

**Valerian tea:** An herb used medicinally as a nerve sedative and antispasmodic.

**Vernix:** A creamy white substance that protects the fetus' skin.

# Suggested Reading List

The following books contain non-fiction and fictional accounts of women's childbearing experiences.

*The Garden of Eros.* Dorothy Bryant. Ata Books, 1979.

*Giving Birth: The Parents' Emotions in Childbirth.* Sheila Kitzinger. Schocken Books, 1978.

*Spiritual Midwifery.* Ina May Gaskin. Book Publishing Company, 1978.

*Birth Stories: The Experience Remembered.* Janet Isaacs Ashford, ed. The Crossing Press, 1984.

*Ever Since Eve: Personal Reflections on Childbirth.* Nancy Caldwell Sorel. Oxford Press, 1984.

*The Mothers' Book: Shared Experiences.* Ronnie Friedland and Carol Kort. Houghton Mifflin Company, 1981.

*A Mother's Journal: A Keepsake Book for Thoughts and Dreams.* Running Press, 1985.

*I Want To Tell You About My Baby.* Roslyn Banish. Wingbow Press, 1982.

*Ended Beginnings: Healing Childbearing Losses.* Claudia Panuthos and Catherine Romeo. Bergin and Garvey Publishers, 1984.

*Artemis Speaks: V.B.A.C. (Vaginal Birth After Cesarean Section) Stories and Natural Childbirth Information.* Nan Koehler. Jerald R. Brown, Inc., 1985.

*Mabel: The Story of One Midwife.* Elizabeth Redditt-Lyon. Red Lyon Publications, 1982. (Out of print)

*Birth Book.* Raven Lang. Genesis Press, 1972. (Out of print)

*A Guide to Midwifery: Heart and Hands.* Elizabeth Davis. Celestial Arts, 1987.